WHAT WIKI DOESN'T WANT *YOU* TO KNOW ABOUT MACROBIOTICS

*100+ Scientific & Medical Studies Showing
the Benefits of a Plant-Based Macrobiotic Diet*

Planetary Health, Inc.

Makropedia.com
Encyclopedia of Diet & Health

What Wikipedia Doesn't Want You to Know About Macrobiotics
By Planetary Health Institute

© 2017 by Planetary Health, Inc.

ISBN 978-1546668428
ISBN 10: 154666842X

Published by Amberwaves Press
PO Box 487, Becket MA 01223
413-623-0012
Makropedia.com

Printed in the U.S.A.

First edition August 2017

Hippocratic Oath Vows to Use Food As Medicine

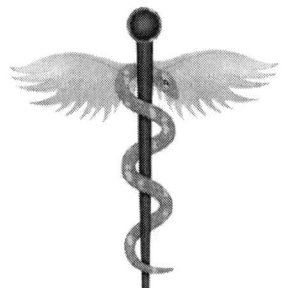

The Hippocratic Oath, composed by Hippocrates, the Father of Medicine, 2500 years ago, pledges to apply "dietetic measures for the benefit of the sick." Modern medicine replaced the food-oriented approach of the original Greek with "do no harm," since modern medicine no longer focuses on diet or nutrition. The original Oath also prohibits the use of deadly drugs, surgery, and other practices that govern healthcare today and which are often unnecessary or harmful:

I swear by Apollo Physician and Asclepius and Hygieia and Panacea and all the gods and goddesses, making them my witnesses, that I will fulfill according to my ability and judgment this oath and this covenant:

To hold him who has taught me this art as equal to my parents and to live my life in partnership with him . . .

I will apply dietetic measures for the benefit of the sick according to my ability and judgment: I will keep them from harm and injustice.

I will neither give a deadly drug to anybody if asked for it, nor will I make a suggestion to this effect. Similarly, I will not give to a woman an abortive remedy. In purity and holiness, I will guard my life and my art.

I will not use the knife, not even on sufferers from stone, but will withdraw in favor of such men as are engaged in this work.

Whatever houses I may visit, I will come for the benefit of the sick, remaining free of all intentional injustice, of all mischief, and in particular of sexual relations with both female and male persons, be they free or slaves.

What I may see or hear in the course of the treatment or even outside of the treatment in regard to the life of men, which on no account one must spread abroad, I will keep to myself holding such things shameful to be spoken about.

If I fulfill this oath and do not violate it, may it be granted to me to enjoy life and art, being honored with fame among all men for all time to come; if I transgress it and swear falsely, may the opposite of all this be my lot.

The translation is from the original Greek in Ancient Medicine: Selected Papers of Ludwig Edelstein, *translated by Owsei Temkin and C. Lilian Temkin (Johns Hopkins University Press, 1961).*

Contents

Hippocratic Oath 3
Preface by Alex Jack 5
Introduction 11
Macrobiotics 13
History 14
Conceptual Basis 18
Dietary Practice 24
Standard Macrobiotic Dietary
  Guidelines 24
Kitchenware 26
Lifestyle Guidelines 26
Natural Healing 29
Scientific and Medical Studies 32
  Ancient Nutrition 32
  Macrobiotic Nutrition 33
  Heart Disease 36
  Cancer 38
    Breast 42
    Colon 43
    Endometrial 45
    Lung 45
    Pancreatic 46
    Prostate 46
    Stomach 47
    General Medical Opinion 48
  AIDS 49
  Arthritis 51
  Autism 53
  Celiac Disease 54
  Children's Health 55
  Crohn's Disease 56
  Diabetes 56
  Ebola 58
  Environmental Illness 59

  Geriatrics 59
  Gluten Intolerance 60
  Hospital Food 61
  Medical Education 62
  Mental and Emotional Health 62
  Microwave Cooking 63
  Migraine and PMS 64
  Nuclear Radiation 64
  Obesity 67
  Osteoporosis 67
  Pregnancy and Childcare 68
Lifestyle 69
  Chewing 69
  Exercise and Fitness 71
  Arts and Culture 71
Social Health 72
  Ancient Food Pattern 72
  Diet and Agriculture 75
  Crime and Violence 76
  Peace and Social Justice 79
Planetary Health 81
  Nutrient Decline 81
  Global Warming 84
  Electromagnetic Fields 84
  Energy and Transmutation 85
  Light Pollution 87
Controversies 88
The Coming Era 89
Appendix: On the Absolute
  Sincerity of Great Physicians 90
Macrobiotic Resources 91
About the Authors 99
References 100

Symbols used in this book:

    Macrobiotic case histories, reports, articles (sheaf of grain)
    Scientific or medical studies, reports, articles (caduceus healing wand)

Preface
What Wikipedia Doesn't Want You to Know about Macrobiotics (and Holistic Health)
By Alex Jack

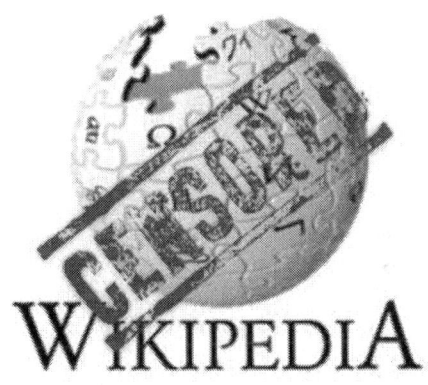

What is macrobiotics? Every day nearly a thousand people look up this term on Wikipedia. It's at the top of the Search list. The opening sentence of the popular online encyclopedia reads: "A macrobiotic diet (or macrobiotics) is a fad diet fixed on ideas about types of food drawn from Zen Buddhism.[1]

The entry proceeds to go downhill from there, claiming there is no medical evidence in support of macrobiotics, following the diet will put you at risk for scurvy, and children may be particularly prone to nutritional deficiencies. All of these claims are outrageous and demonstrably false. So is the basic premise that the macrobiotic way of eating is a fad diet or a way of thinking derived from Zen.

In actuality, macrobiotics is humanity's oldest dietary pattern, dating to the emergence of our species by eating foraged grains and vegetables—about 4 million years ago, according to the most recent scientific studies (*Proceedings of the National Academy of Sciences*, 2013) and mastering the use of fire for cooking. This is hardly a fad! The modern way of eating, high in saturated fat, dairy protein, refined sugar, and other processed foods, is the real fad diet—dating to only a hundred years or more.

The Greek word μακροβιοσ (macrobios), from which the concept *macrobiotics* originated, was coined by Hippocrates, in the 5th century BCE. The Father of Medicine used the word to mean "long life," and along with *macrobii, macrobian*, and other variants, it entered the Classical and Renaissance vocabulary to refer to healthy, long-lived peoples. Like Hippocrates, whose approach to health and healing is summed up in a proverb widely attributed to him "Let food be thy medicine and medicine be thy food," most followers of macrobiotics through the ages observed a balanced plant-based diet with little if any animal food.

As for Zen, it is true that adherents of this Buddhist sect ate in a semi-macrobiotic way until modern times. But then so did Buddhists of other schools, as did Jews, Zoroastrians, Gnostics, Christians, Muslims, Taoists, Confucians, Africans, Native Americans, and people from many other faiths and cultures. It would

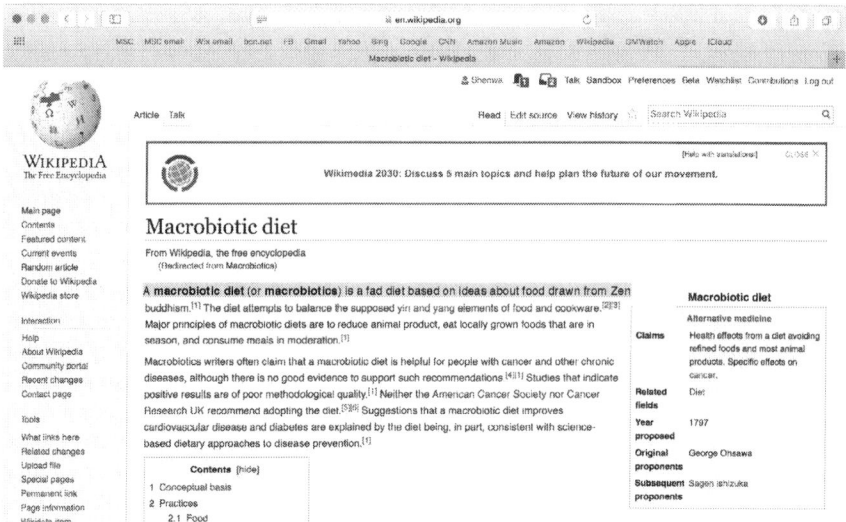

be more accurate for Wikipedia to say that macrobiotics is a diet drawn from Jesus and his followers (who ate primarily grains, vegetables, fruit, and a little fish) than from Zen. But that claim too, however true, is much too narrow a perspective. Macrobiotics is a universal concept and practice. As educator Michio Kushi observed, "It is not the limited philosophy of one time or place, one country or people, one teacher or organization, one religion or way of life. It is universal in its scope and eternal in its duration."[2]

Reading the Wikipedia article transported me back to the late 1960s and early 1970s. During the hippie and counterculture era, Dr. Frederick Stare, chairman of the nutrition department at Harvard University wrote a lurid article on macrobiotics "The Diet That's Killing Our Kids" for *Ladies Home Journal*, the nation's foremost women's magazine. During that era—the nutritional dark ages when the Basic Four food groups (two of which were meat and dairy) reigned and a nation of hamburger and hot dog lovers was bombing the rice fields of Southeast Asia to smithereens—the FDA and FBI raided macrobiotic centers and natural foods stores, and the medical profession ridiculed vegetarian diets as harmful and deficient—if not politically subversive.

Thankfully, times changed, even if Wikipedia remains stuck in a time warp—a dark era when the Standard American Diet was not yet linked to heart disease, cancer, and diabetes. That came in 1977 with the historic U.S. Senate Report *Dietary Goals for the United States* associating the modern way of eating with six of the ten leading causes of death. Studies on macrobiotics at Harvard Medical School, Framingham Heart Study, National Institutes of Health, CDC, and other top medical organizations, as well as statements by the American Medical Association, the American Cancer Society, and other medical societies, later confirmed the health benefits of macrobiotics, and the Kushis' were honored with a Permanent Collection on Macrobiotics at the National Museum of American History as the new millennium arrived. On the basis of scores of peer-reviewed studies on the benefits of macrobiotics, the medical committee of the Smithsonian created the collection. The U.S. House of Representatives passed a resolution unanimously honoring the Kushis and the macrobiotic community.

Yet none of this appears in Wikipedia. With a view to setting the record straight in "the encyclopedia that anyone can edit," I revised and updated the entry on "Macrobiotic Diet," carefully including all the citations in the *New England Journal of Medicine, Atherosclerosis, American Journal of Clinical Nutrition,* and the other peer-reviewed journals.

Within minutes, before I had completed uploading my revisions, my computer screen froze and a message appeared that my entry was blocked! It turned out that an administrator had intervened, deleted all my updates, and reverted to the original pejorative entry. A message on the editor's page said that my inserts were "fringe promo" and had been deleted. A cursory look at previous edits on the "View History" tab showed a pattern of attempts by other citizen editors to bring the article up to date, and each time they were rejected as biased and redundant.

Curious, I discovered that the embattled guardian of public health and nutritional morals was Alex Brown, a medical editor, who proudly notes in a link to his bio that he was once named "one of the top 10 medical contributors" to Wikipedia. The other articles he created on Wikipedia included "List of Ineffective Cancer Treatments," "Pseudomedicine," and—believe it or not—"Frederick J. Stare."

As Max Planck, who introduced the concept of the paradigm shift, famously observed, "A new scientific truth does not triumph by convincing its opponents and making them see the light, but rather because its opponents eventually die, and a new generation grows up that is familiar with it."[3] It seems Dr. Stare is the exception that proves the rule. Like a vengeful ghost in Shakespeare, he has come back from the bardo to hijack macrobiotics' digital identity!

From the adulatory write up of Dr. Stare on Wikipedia you would hardly realize his career ended in disgrace when he was unmasked as a paid consultant to the sugar lobby, junk food cereal companies, and even Big Tobacco! Talk about the diet that's killing our kids! On his kudos page, we learn that Alex Brown received a virtual Cheeseburger, Brownie, and Cup of Coffee for his trolling efforts by fellow Wikipedian administrators. I rest my case.

Actually, macrobiotics is not being singled out on Wikipedia, and I shouldn't take its antebellum nutritional stance so personally. The entries for Homeopathy, Acupuncture, Reiki, and other holistic approaches are even worse! It is mindboggling that in a time when virtually every hospital in the country has integrated acupuncture and therapeutic touch into its medical practice that Wikipedia claims there is no evidence that they work!

When I mentioned my frustration to fellow writer and researcher Bill Shurtleff, he laughed at my naiveté. He characterized Wikipedia as a battlefield for contested ideologies and vested interests. He said that whenever he attempted to add a

citation from *The Book of Miso, The Book of Tofu*, and other classics that he co-authored or list his Soyinfo Center, the world's most comprehensive online database on soybeans and soyfoods, his reference was deleted. He is now permanently blacklisted from the site. Instead of Wikipedia, he recommends using *Encyclopedia Britannica*, which relies on seasoned authorities, not self-appointed guardians of nutritional and medical correctness.

As I later discovered, thousands of people signed a petition on Change.org to halt Wikipedia's attacks on holistic and alternative medicine: "Wikipedia is widely used and trusted. Unfortunately, much of the information related to holistic approaches to healing is biased, misleading, out-of-date, and just plain wrong." The petition went on to say that for five years repeated efforts to correct the misinformation were blocked. In response to this appeal, Wikipedia's co-founder Jimmy Wales scoffed that there was no place for "the work of lunatic charlatans." As other independent investigators concluded, "The information on Wikipedia is filtered to remove any talk of natural remedies, natural cures, and organic medicine, referring to anything that is not lab-made as quack medicine, anti-science, or even conspiracy theory when it challenges 'science-based' information that has no independent research sourcing. The information that makes it through the Wikipedia filters and is published is pure mainstream, allopathic, and biotechnology driven."[4] Mike Bundraft, a Neuro-Linguistic Programming expert, launched a Kickstarter campaign to publish *Un•Biased: The Truth About the Healing Arts on Wikipedia*, because of the site's hatchet job on dozens of alternative approaches. Many schools and colleges, as well as news sites, bar their students or teachers from using Wikipedia for research papers or articles on account of its slanted viewpoints, fake history, and rampant sexism (85% of editors are male).[5]

Articles on genetic engineering in Wikipedia also whitewash the dangers of GMOs and falsely claim there is a broad scientific consensus on their safety. This is absurd. *Consumers Reports,* the largest independent product safety magazine in the country, has long questioned the safety of GMOs, and virtually every major health and environmental organization from the Sierra Club to the National Audubon Society have expressed deep concern. Many medical organizations support mandatory labeling and strict oversight, including the American Public Health Association, the American Association of Environmental Medicine, American Nursing Association, American College of Physicians, the California Medical Association, and the British Medical Association.

[Screenshot of Wikipedia article "Genetically modified food controversies"]

After I told my colleagues at Planetary Health about this experience, we decided to publish our own entry on macrobiotics as a small book and link it on our web sites. Hence this volume. Whether it is balanced and fair, biased or unbiased, we leave to each reader to decide. But it does include vital information summarizing over 100 scientific studies, medical reports, and case histories that an informed public has the right to know about. We suspect that a high percentage of online searches for macrobiotics—as well as homeopathy, Reiki, acupuncture, yoga, and other holistic approaches—are inspired by medical doctors and other healthcare professionals who recommend complementary alternatives to their patients.

Denying the public safe, simple, effective, commonsense remedies and potentially life-saving information is tragic. Such censorship is practicing quack medicine of the worst kind. Even Dr. Stare changed his tune. In an interview with the *New York Times* in 1978 following the release of the landmark *Dietary Goals for the United States*, he told the *New York Times*: 'As I see the [macrobiotic] diet today, it is really not much more than a typical vegetarian diet. Anybody switching from the average American diet to a macrobiotic diet is going to take off 10 or 15 pounds, just by reducing his fat intake.'"[6]

The truth has never stayed silenced for long. History will judge whether macrobiotics, holistic health, and the whole trend of modern society, including the medical profession, to embrace a sane food and agricultural system based on organic, plant-based foods is a fad diet or the key to reconnecting with humanity's ancestral roots and creating a healthy, peaceful, sustainable future.

Makropedia.com

> Makro • pédia | Comprehensive online reference work for creating personal and planetary health, especially through dietary awareness and practice [from Greek *makrobios* whole, long, or great life + Latin *paideia* education]

Ten years ago, when I was living in Amsterdam, I worked with Adelbert Nelissen and other colleagues at the Kushi Institute of Europe to create Makropedia.com, an online encyclopedia on diet and health. Our goal was to make freely and universally available vital information on food, cooking, and healing to students, parents, workers, farmers, doctors and nurses, and people of all backgrounds and orientations in Africa, the Middle East, Asia, Latin America, and worldwide. We hoped the new web site (initially in English and then in other languages) would eventually include video clips (e.g., how to cook grains and vegetables), webinars, and interactive charts and displays. At that time, we faced some of the same problems with Wikipedia, Google, and other online sites and search engines that were hostile or indifferent toward plant-based diets and alternative medicine. Unfortunately, Adelbert passed away a few years ago and the project remained dormant.

However, after this most recent experience with Wikipedia, we feel it is time to revive and introduce Makropedia. In the months ahead, under the auspices of Planetary Health, Inc., our nonprofit educational organization, we plan to launch Makropedia.com. The first entry or article will be the contents of this book documenting the benefits of macrobiotics and allied plant-based approaches to health and well being. After that, we plan to post an A–Z listing of informative articles on holistic principles and practices, dietary and way of life guidelines, menus and recipes, case histories and community accounts, home remedies, nutritional information and food composition tables, meridian charts, and a wealth of other material that is not readily accessible.

We invite your support and participation in this special project. Visit Makropedia.com, monitor our progress, become part of the team, and contribute your knowledge and experience.

Alex Jack, president of Planetary Health, Inc., is a macrobiotic teacher, counselor, and author. He has served as editor-in-chief of East West Journal, *executive director of Kushi Institute, and director of the One Peaceful World Society. His books include* The Cancer-Prevention Diet *with Michio Kushi (St. Martin's Press, 3rd edition, 2010),* The Macrobiotic Path to Total Health *with Michio Kushi (Ballantine Books, 2003),* Aveline Kushi's Complete Guide to Macrobiotic Cooking *(Time-Warner Books, 1985), annotated editions and commentaries on* Hamlet *and* As You Like It *(Amberwaves Press, 2005, 2012), and* The One Peaceful World Cookbook: 150 Vegan Macrobiotic Recipes for Vibrant Health & Happiness *with Sachi Kato (BenBella Books, 2017).*

Introduction

"Let food be thy medicine, and thy medicine be food." —Hippocrates

During the last half century, macrobiotics has been in the forefront of the health and diet revolution, serving as the catalyst for many of the dietary and lifestyle changes now circling the globe. Macrobiotics has introduced modern societies to organically grown whole foods and naturally processed foods, including brown rice, whole wheat, and other whole grains; miso, tofu, tempeh, and other traditional soy products; a cornucopia of fresh garden vegetables; wakame, kombu, and other sea vegetables; and a variety of high-quality seasonings, condiments, and sugar- and dairy-free desserts and snacks. Macrobiotics has also popularized holistic health, self-healing, and alternative and complementary methods that are now embraced by millions of people and by the medical profession.

"Macrobiotics" comes from *makrobios*, the Greek term for "Long Life" and "Great Life." Hippocrates, the Father of Medicine, coined the word, and in the modern era it has been developed by Michio and Aveline Kushi and other educators in North America, South America, Europe, Asia, Africa, and the Middle East. By creating our minds and bodies from whole natural foods in a spirit of thankfulness, we can contribute to personal health, social well being, and planetary health and peace.

The benefits of a macrobiotic diet are widely recognized today, as the scientific and medical studies and other accounts in this guide show. From a tiny seed in the 1960s, macrobiotic principles have blossomed into a tree of life, nourishing society at many levels. The landmark dietary and nutritional changes over the last generation have been influenced and shaped by macrobiotics, from *Dietary Goals for the United States,* the landmark report by a Select U.S. Senate Committee in the late 1970s to the government's Food Guide Pyramid in the 1980s, from the creation of the Office of Alternative Medicine within the National Institutes of Health (NIH) in the 1990s to the shift toward a plant-centered diet and vegan cuisine in the 2000s.

The momentous changes that took place constitute a nutritional axis shift. The Basic Four food groups—based on meat and dairy food—were replaced with a more balanced way of eating centered on grains, vegetables, fruits, and other plant foods. As the new century began, the *U.S. Dietary Guidelines* accompanying the Food Guide Pyramid called upon Americans to "use plant foods as the foundation of your meals":

There are many ways to create a healthy eating pattern, but they all start with the three food groups at the base of the Pyramid: grains, fruits, and vegetables. Eating a variety of grains (especially whole grain foods), fruits, and vegetables is the basis of healthy eating. Enjoy meals that have rice, pasta, tortillas, or whole grain bread as the center of the plate. . . . Eating plenty of whole grains, such as whole grain bread or oatmeal, as part of the healthful eating patterns described by these guidelines, may help protect you against many chronic diseases.[7]

The benefits of a macrobiotic way of eating have been recognized by the major scientific and medical societies and published in leading journals, including the *New England Journal of Medicine, Journal of the American Medical Association, American Journal of Clinical Nutrition, Lancet,* and dozens of others. In a recent cover story on heart health, *Consumer Reports,* the largest public interest magazine in the country, called on its millions of readers to "Redesign Your Plate" and make whole grains, beans, vegetables, fruits, seeds and nuts "the centerpieces of your meals" and "think of meat as a condiment."[8]

This book, part of a new series on Macrobiotic Principles & Practices, includes an introduction to macrobiotics, a brief history, conceptual basis, dietary and lifestyle guidelines, daily menu and recipes, and a summary of this vast body of professional research, insight, and understanding. The citation for each listing follows at the end for further reference. Original articles are available at many medical libraries and, in a growing number of cases, online. Abstracts for medical studies are available on Medline at www.pubmed.gov.

The studies were primarily designed to evaluate the effects of a macrobiotic way of eating. Some early studies labeled practitioners as "strict vegetarians," and, as it enters the mainstream, a macrobiotic diet is now often referred to in medical literature as simply a "plant-based diet." Besides peer-reviewed studies, we have included selected individual case history reports (most of which are the subject of published books or articles), hypotheses by macrobiotic teachers and counselors on the origin and cause of AIDS, Ebola, the BRCA gene mutation, Celiac disease, gluten sensitivity, and other emerging plagues and disorders, and several key dietary or lifestyle studies related to planetary health. Finally, there is a section at the end with information on macrobiotic education, food companies, publications, and other essential resources.

We are grateful to the many researchers, teachers, counselors, cooks, farmers, seaweed harvesters, natural foods manufacturers and distributors, parents and children, and others who make up the macrobiotic community. Together, they are helping to create a new model of diet and health that is transforming the planet.

Alex Jack, Edward Esko, and Bettina Zumdick
The Berkshires

The authors are macrobiotic teachers, counselors, and founders of Planetary Health, Inc., a 501 (c) 3 nonprofit that sponsors the Macrobiotic Wellness Retreat and Macrobiotic Summer Conference.

Macrobiotics

Macrobiotics is the art of living a bright, healthy, peaceful life. It encompasses a deep understanding of humanity's origin and destiny, natural order, and the cosmos. It encompasses evolution and history, climate and environment, anatomy and physiology, behavior and activity, thoughts and emotions, relationships and communities, arts and cultures, science and medicine, societies and civilizations, and consciousness and spiritual development.

A macrobiotic diet and lifestyle is grounded in a way of eating centered on whole grains and other primarily plant-based foods and on living in harmony and balance with nature and the infinite universe. It embraces all complementary opposites, including East and West, North and South, traditional and modern, material and spiritual, visionary and practical, and strives to create a peaceful mind, home, and world community.[9]

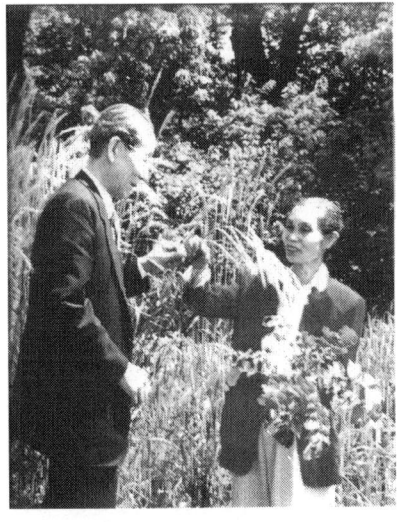

Michio and Aveline Kushi, leaders of the modern macrobiotic movement

The macrobiotic movement, led by educators Michio Kushi (1926-2014) and his wife Aveline Kushi (1923-2001), pioneered the natural foods movement, organic farming, and alternative healing beginning in the 1960s and over the last half century spearheaded the historical shift in modern society from an animal- to a plant-based diet.[10] During this time, macrobiotics has been studied by the National Institutes of Health (NIH), CDC (Center for Disease Control and Prevention), Harvard Medical School, Framingham Heart Study, and other scientific and medical organizations.[11]

Its positive benefits in helping to prevent and relieve high blood pressure, high cholesterol, and heart disease; selected cancers, diabetes; immune-deficiency diseases; and other chronic conditions have been published in the *New England Journal of Medicine, American Journal of Clinical Nutrition, Lancet, Nutrition and Cancer,* and other peer-reviewed journals. As *The American Medical Association Family Medical Guide* concluded: "In general, the macrobiotic diet is a healthful way of eating."[12]

The Smithsonian Institution recognized the contribution of macrobiotics to "healthy diet, our increasingly global culture, alternative healing, peace studies, and traditions of grassroots activism" with the creation of a permanent Michio and Aveline Kushi Collection at the National Museum of American History in

Washington, D.C. in 1998.[13] The macrobiotic community today continues to be on the cutting edge of personal and planetary change with a global network of thousands of teachers, counselors, and chefs, as well as educational centers, communities, organic farms, natural foods companies, restaurants, businesses, small publishers, and social media.

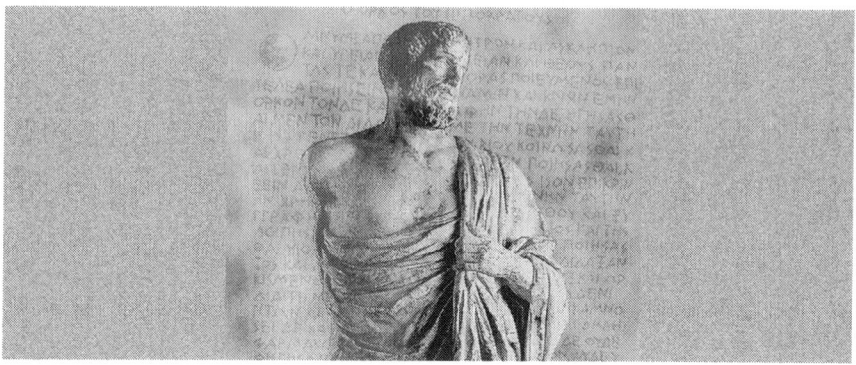

Hippocrates, the Father of Medicine, coined the term macrobios (long life) about 2500 years ago

History

Macrobiotics is based on an understanding and application of the universal laws of change and harmony that govern body, mind, and spirit, as well as nature, society, and the cosmos. The concept goes back to Hippocrates, the Father of Medicine, who used μακροβιοσ (*makrobios*) meaning "long life," in the 5th century BCE and had a dietary approach to healing, centered on barley, wheat, millet, and other whole grains.[14]

As Michio Kushi explained in of *The Book of Macrobiotics: The Universal Way of Health, Happiness, and Peace* (2013): "Macrobiotics is the collective wisdom and universal heritage of humanity. Macrobiotics is not the manifestation, property, or exclusive possession of a single era, culture, society, nation, religion, school, family, or individual."[15] From ancient times, macrobiotic teachings flourished in ancient China, India, Africa, the Middle East, Europe, and, the Americas.

In the mid-1960s, the Kushis began teaching in Boston, started Erewhon Trading Company, the pioneer natural foods store, and popularized the Standard Macrobiotic Diet consisting of organically grown whole grains and grain products such as brown rice and whole wheat bread and pasta; miso and others soups; beans and bean products such as tofu and tempeh; vegetables from land and sea; and sugar- and dairy-free desserts and snacks.[16] Animal food, especially fish and seafood, was optional, and many followers are vegan.[17] In the late 1960s and early 1970s, macrobiotics spread along with the rise of the counterculture, yoga, meditation, and the peace movement.

In his lectures about the war in Vietnam, Michio Kushi contrasted the simple grain-and-vegetable diet of Southeast Asia with the heavy meat-and-sugar based diet of the United States and Soviet Union and warned that the modern way of eating was contributing not only to heart disease, cancer, and other degenerative conditions but also to a narrow fixed mentality, mood swings, violence, and war. As the spearhead of the natural foods movement, macrobiotic food companies included Muso, Lima Foods, Manna, Eden Foods, Mitoku, Chico-San, Westbrae, South River Miso, and many others.

Initially, the plant-based macrobiotic dietary approach was so different from the standard modern diet and appealed to hippies, peaceniks, and others who had opted out of modern society that it was misunderstood, ridiculed, and attacked in scientific and medical quarters as nutritionally deficient.[18] The FDA raided macrobiotic centers and health food stores, and Dr. Frederick J. Stare, chairman of the department of nutrition at Harvard University School of Public Health warned against "The Diet That's Killing Our Kids" in *Ladies Home Journal*.[19]

MONTHLY, WEEKLY, and DAILY CONSUMPTION

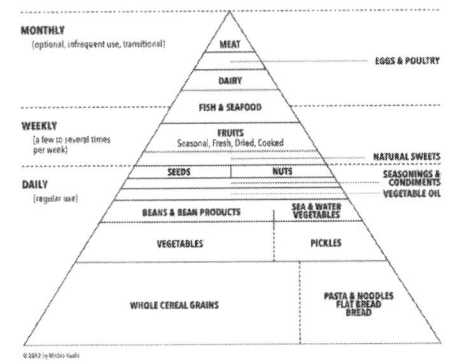

MONTHLY (optional, infrequent use, transitional)
- MEAT
- EGGS & POULTRY
- DAIRY
- FISH & SEAFOOD

WEEKLY (a few to several times per week)
- FRUITS — Seasonal, Fresh, Dried, Cooked
- NATURAL SWEETS
- SEEDS
- NUTS
- SEASONINGS & CONDIMENTS
- VEGETABLE OIL

DAILY (regular use)
- BEANS & BEAN PRODUCTS
- SEA & WATER VEGETABLES
- VEGETABLES
- PICKLES
- WHOLE CEREAL GRAINS
- PASTA & NOODLES, FLAT BREAD, BREAD

© 2012 by Michio Kushi

DAILY FOOD CONSUMPTION

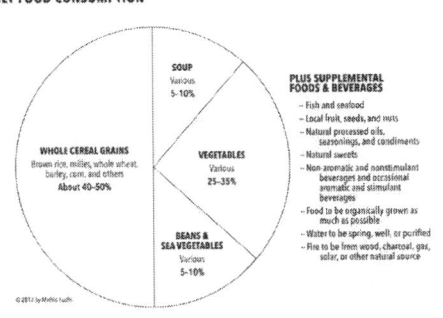

- SOUP — Various, 5–10%
- VEGETABLES — Various, 25–35%
- WHOLE CEREAL GRAINS — Brown rice, millet, whole wheat, barley, corn, and others — About 40–50%
- BEANS & SEA VEGETABLES — Various, 5–10%

PLUS SUPPLEMENTAL FOODS & BEVERAGES
- Fish and seafood
- Local fruit, seeds, and nuts
- Natural processed oils, seasonings, and condiments
- Natural sweets
- Non-aromatic and nonstimulant beverages and occasional aromatic and stimulant beverages
- Food to be organically grown as much as possible
- Water to be spring, well, or purified
- Fire to be from wood, charcoal, gas, solar, or other natural source

© 2012 by Michio Kushi

Within several years, society's attitude toward low-fat, vegetarian, and vegan diets began to change. The Senate Select Committee on Nutrition and Human Needs released *Dietary Goals for the United States* in 1977 warning of an unrecognized "wave of overnutrition" and linking six of the ten leading causes of death to the modern way of eating.[20] In the early 1990s, the Food Guide Pyramid (with grains forming the foundation of a healthy daily way of eating) replaced the Basic Four food groups (the previous model high in animal quality protein). The integrity of Dr. Stare of Harvard was questioned when it emerged he was a paid consultant to the food industry and had sought tobacco company funding. Following these momentous changes, macrobiotics began to attract favorable interest among leading scientific and medical organizations. From being labeled as a dangerous, fad diet and a pseudoscience, macrobiotics was increasingly viewed as a model for better health and well-being.

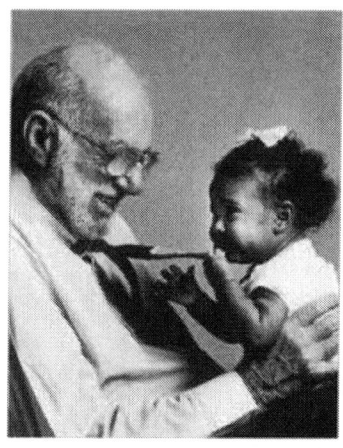

Dr. Benjamin Spock promoted macrobiotics toward the end of his life

Dr. Benjamin Spock, described by the *New York Times* as "the most influential pediatrician of all time," followed a macrobiotic way of eating during the last decade of his life.[21] In the final edition of his book, *Baby and Child Care*, released just weeks after his death at age 94 in 1998, he recommended that children be brought up on a plant-based diet.

"When parents offer healthy foods—vegetables, fruits, whole grains, and beans—at home, and when the whole family, including the parents, makes these foods front and center in the diet, children learn tastes that can help them throughout life."[22] Within two weeks of starting macrobiotics himself and discontinuing dairy foods, Dr. Spock noted in his book, "My chronic bronchitis went away after years of unsuccessful antibiotic treatments."

Over the years, the Kushis and their educational organizations—the East West Foundation and Kushi Institute—inspired scores of medical studies, beginning with Harvard Medical School in the early 1970s, that documented the benefits of the macrobiotic approach in lowering cholesterol and blood pressure; preventing or relieving heart disease, selected cancers, and diabetes; and improving the quality of life and well-being of children, families, and the elderly.[23] The Second International Conference on Dietary Assessment Methods, a large gathering of six hundred medical researchers sponsored by the Harvard School of Public Health and the World Health Organization, featured a macrobiotic banquet at the John F. Kennedy Library in Boston. Michio Kushi led a WHO conference on AIDS in the Republic of the Congo for several hundred physicians and native healers. Macrobiotics also helped to reduce aggression and anti-social behavior among juvenile inmates, assist in the rehabilitation of prisoners, and contribute to reconciliation and harmony among opposing religious and ethnic groups in war-torn regions of the world.[24]

In 2002, an expert panel convened by the National Cancer Institute (NCI) voted unanimously to approve clinical trials of the macrobiotic approach to cancer based on a National Institutes of Health (NIH) Best Case Study of 77 individuals who recovered from a variety of malignancies with the help of macrobiotics.[25] Subsequent medical tests, and reports from the Methodist Hospital in Philadelphia, Holy Redeemer Hospital in Meadowbrook, Penn., Tulane University, M.D. Anderson Cancer Center at the University of Texas in Houston, National Tumor Institute in Milan, Italy, and Moores Cancer Center, University of California, San Diego found that the macrobiotic diet was instrumental in preventing or relieving tumors, including those of the breast, prostate, pancreas, lungs, and other organs.[26] The macrobiotic approach has also been helpful in relieving radiation sickness, from the atomic bombings in Japan to the nuclear accidents in the Soviet Union.[27]

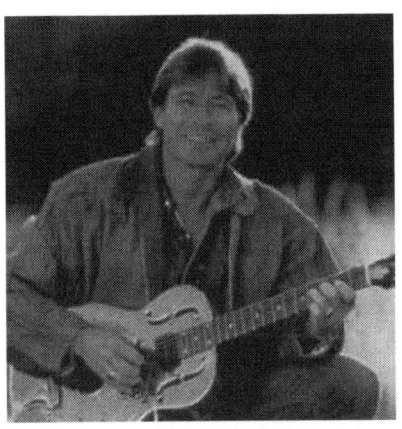

Singer John Denver gave several benefit concerts for macrobiotics

From the communes and health food stores of the 1960s and 1970s to the spas and wellness centers of the 1980s and 1990s, macrobiotics began to move into the mainstream. The Ritz Carlton and Prince Hotel chains started serving macrobiotic food to their international guests. The Kellogg School of Management at Northwestern University established a dining room with macrobiotic entrées for busy executives taking seminars and macrobiotic teachers and cooks were invited to the White House, Capitol Hill, and the United Nations.[28] Macrobiotics was profiled in *Vogue, New York Times, Boston Globe*, and other leading publications, and Bill Dufty, John Lennon, Yoko Ono, Barbra Streisand, John Travolta, Sarah Jessica Parker, Madonna, Gwyneth Paltrow, Steven Seagal, Andie MacDowell, Nicole Kidman, Tom Cruise, Sting, Boy George, Julia Roberts, Alicia Silverstone, Rachel Weisz, Guy Richie, Kim Kardashian, and other celebrities had their own macrobiotic chefs. Actress Gloria Swanson and singer John Denver were particularly vocal in supporting macrobiotics, often appearing with the Kushis at macrobiotic events and fundraising concerts.[29]

In establishing a permanent Kushi collection at the National Museum of American History in Washington, D.C., Spencer Crew, the museum director, noted: "The National Museum of American History at the Smithsonian Institution is honored to present the [Special] Collection on Macrobiotics and Alternative Health

Care. This collection of health, nutrition, and personal family materials and artifacts documents important and little studied aspects of American life and culture. ... The significance of macrobiotics in American life is little understood although it relates to such broad historical issues as the postwar move toward a more healthy diet, our increasingly global culture, alternative healing, peace studies, and traditions of grassroots activism."[30]

On the initiative of Rep. Dennis Kucinich (Dem., Ohio), the U.S. House of Representatives passed a resolution unanimously honoring the Kushis for their dedication and contribution to the nation's health and well-being.[31]

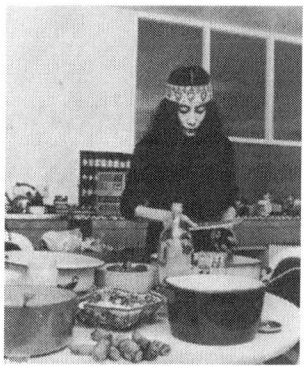

Yoko Ono cooking with John Lennon in England. They took macrobiotic cooking classes and met with the Kushis in Boston

Imagine all the people living life in peace, you
You may say I'm a dreamer
But I'm not the only one
I hope some day you'll join us
And the world will be as one . . .
—John Lennon, Imagine

Conceptual Basis

Macrobiotics is based on creating balance and harmony with nature and the cosmos. The universal laws of change and harmony were studied, applied, and celebrated by all traditional cultures and societies, forming the universal foundation for the world's intellectual, social, cultural, philosophical, religious, and spiritual traditions.[32] The way to embody this order in daily life was taught by sages, poets, and artists, including Homer, Moses, Buddha, Lao Tzu, Confucius, Jesus, Mohammad, Dante, Hildegard of Bingen, Shakespeare, Steiner, Gandhi, and Martin Luther King, Jr. Under many names and forms this order has been rediscovered, applied, and taught for thousands of years. It is inscribed in the Bible, Upanishads, I Ching, Yellow Emperor's Classic, Tao Te Ching, Bhagavad Gita, Hippocratic writings, Qur'an, and other sacred texts and scriptures.[33]

As Kushi explained, "The infinite universe is a paradise full of joy and peace. It is without beginning and without end. It is spaceless and timeless. However, because it is moving in all dimensions at infinite speed it creates phenomena that are infinitesimal and ephemeral. These manifestations have a beginning and an end, a front and a back, measure and duration, and may be viewed as forms appearing and disappearing in an ocean of cosmic energy."[34]

The infinite universe, or the creative source known as God in some traditions, though itself invisible and beyond the apprehension of the senses, differentiates into two antagonistic and complementary tendencies of centrifugality and centripetality —expansion and contraction, space and time, beginning and end, yin and yang. At the intersection of these two forces, numerous spirals are produced in every dimension.

All phenomena are spirallic in nature, regardless of whether they are visible or invisible, spiritual or physical, energetic or material. Many of the spirals arising in the infinite ocean of existence appear manifest to our eyes. The physical universe, stretching over ten billion light years in every direction and itself spirallic in structure, contains billions of spiral galaxies, some hundreds of thousands of light years in diameter, which periodically appear and disappear. In turn, these galaxies contain hundreds of millions of spirallic solar systems.

In each spirallic solar system, various planets, together with millions of comets, are spiralling around the spirallic center called the sun. Each planet receives a charge of incoming, centripetal force towards its center—a spirallic energy we call gravity. Meanwhile, as a result of turning on its axis, an outgoing, centrifugal force is generated toward the periphery. Together these two forces combine to keep the planet in orbit about the sun.

On earth, a small planet within a solar system belonging to the spiral galaxy called the Milky Way, centripetal force and centrifugal force produce unaccountable phenomena that appear and disappear, changing constantly. These planetary phenomena include invisibly minute spirals such as electrons, protons, and other subatomic particles; various kinds of elements that combine to form organic and inorganic compounds; and numerous kinds of botanical and zoological life, including human beings, which appeared during the most recent era of biological evolution on the planet.

As all life exists within worlds of multiple spirals, human life is also spirally constituted and governed. Not only individual human lives but also human history as a whole is subject to the laws of spirallic motion and change. The two antagonistic and complementary forces govern the development of human affairs, underlying patterns of growth and decay, health and sickness, peace and war.

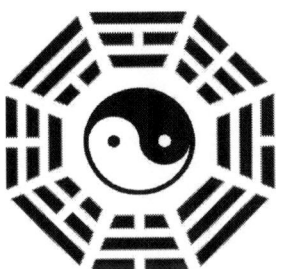

Yin Yang symbol surrounded by the 8 trigrams of the I Ching or Book of Change

Pay heed to the providing of nourishment and to what a person seeks to fill his or her own mouth with. —I Ching

In the Far East, the Tao, or ultimate reality, gives rise to these twin tendencies known as yin and yang. Yang, or heaven's force, manifests as the inward moving centripetal energy coming to the earth from the sun, moon, planets, stars, distant galaxies, and infinite cosmos. Yin, or earth's force, appears as the upward, outward moving centrifugal force arising from the center of the earth and spiraling into the cosmos. These two forces give rise to all plants, animals, and human beings on our planet and throughout the universe.

In the ancient Indian philosophy of Vedanta, underlying Hinduism, this understanding is expressed as Brahman, or the absolute, differentiating into Shiva and Parvati, Krishna and Radha, and other pairs of primordial male and female deities.

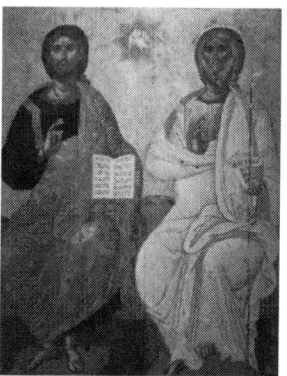

In Thomas's Gospel, Jesus teaches the unity of opposites

In the Gospel According to Thomas, Jesus is asked to explain his teaching and says to his disciples, "If they ask you 'What is the sign of your Father in you?' say to them: 'It is a movement and a rest.'"[35] Throughout this gospel, discovered in Egypt in 1945, Jesus uses complementary opposite energies. In both Thomas and the New Testament, these polarities include heaven and earth, first and last, body and soul, living and dead, flesh and spirit, hidden and revealed, serpent and dove, tree and and fruit, mote and beam.[36]

In Greek mythology, the cosmos was viewed as the eternal field of play of two forces, Love (φιλότης or *Philia*) and Strife (νεῖκος or *Neikos*).[37] Besides Hippocrates, other classical authors, including Herodotus, Aristotle, Galen, and Lucian used the term *makrobios*.[38] Their worldview was shaped by the Four Elements (Earth, Air, Water, and Fire) that was similar to the Five Transformations in Eastern thought and the Five Trees in Paradise in the Gospel According to Thomas. (The quintessence, or fifth element, was often added in Western thought to the Four Elements.)[39]

In early Western literature, the term *macrobios* and its variants—*macrobiote, macrobiosis,* and *macrobian*—became synonymous with a natural way of life centered on whole grains and vegetables. The concept may go back to the Ἄβιοι (abioi) "most just of men," mentioned in the *Iliad* who abstained from war and enjoyed a life of sanctity.[40] The Ethiopians, Thessalians, Biblical patriarchs such as Abraham, and other long-lived people were described as exemplifying *macrobios*. During the Renaissance, Rabelais, the French humanist, includes Macraeon Island of long life in *Gargantua and Pantagruel*, his satire on the follies of society.[41]

During the Enlightenment, the concept found a proponent in Christoph Wilhelm Hufeland, an eighteenth century German philosopher, professor of medicine, and physician to Goethe and the King of Prussia. Going against the scientific tide, he promoted the superiority of a simple plant-based diet, warned against the hazards of eating meat, sugar, and dairy food, and promoted breastfeeding, running, and vigorous exercise, as well as self-healing.

Makrobiotic oder die Kunst, das menschliche Leben zu verlangern ["Macrobiotic or the Art of Prolonging Life"], his most Famous book, appeared in German in 1796 and was the first book to use the term *macrobiotic*:

"The life of man, physically considered, is a peculiar chemico-animal operation; a phenomenon effected by a concurrence of the united powers of Nature with matter in a continual state of change. This, like every other physical operation, must have its defined laws, boundaries, and duration. . . By laying down just principles respecting its essence and wants, and by attending to observations made from experience, the circumstances under which this process may be hastened and shortened, or retarded and prolonged, can be discovered. Upon this may be founded dietetic rules and a medical mode of treatment for preserving life; and hence arises a particular science, the MACROBIOTIC, or the art of prolonging it, which form the subject of the present work."[42]

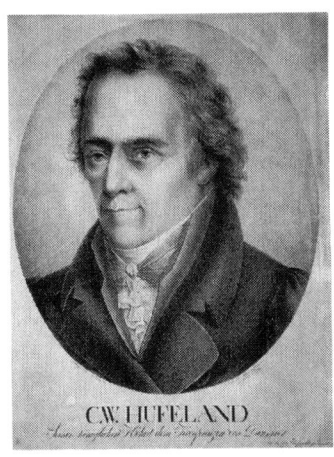

Christoph W. Hufeland, M.D., a German physician, wrote *Macrobiotic or The Art of Prolonging Life* in 1796

Hufeland's book was widely translated, and the concept of macrobiotics appeared in medical lexicons and ordinary dictionaries throughout the 19th and early 20th centuries. In the U.S., the earliest mention is in the *Encyclopedia Americana* in 1838.[43] Sir Richard Burton, translator of the *Arabian Nights* and *Kama Sutra*, set out on a quest for the Bedouin heirs of the ancient *macrobians* whom Herodotus mentions in his travels in sub-Sahara Africa.[44]

In 1908, Sir Norman Lockyer, the discoverer of helium and a Nobel Prize winner, used the term in an article in *Nature*: "The summary of a long list of germinative tests show that a large number of leguminous seeds are macrobiotic, that is, they maintain their vitality for a long period."[45] Dr. Edmond Szekeley wrote a chapter on macrobiotics in a volume on ancient wisdom.[46]

Broadly, other dialectical thinkers in the West who introduced complementary opposite energies as the basis of their approach included Hegel and Marx (*thesis* and *antithesis*), Freud (*ego* and *id* and *libido* and *thanatos*), and Toynbee, who in his *Study of History*, explained that his understanding originated from a study of yin and yang: "Of the various symbols in which different observers in different societies have expressed the activity in the rhythm of the Universe, Yin and Yang are the most apt, because they convey the measure of the rhythm directly and not through some metaphor derived from psychology or mechanics of mathematics. We will therefore use these Sinic symbols in this study henceforward."[47]

In his encyclopedic *Science and Civilization in China*, Joseph Needham describes the ancient art of health and longevity—in both East and West—as *macrobiotics* and in China identified it primarily with Taoist immortality practices.[48]

In the East, macrobiotic forerunners include Ekiken Kaibara (1630-1714), a Japanese physician who recommended a balanced diet to protect against chronic disease. "A person should prefer light, simple meals. One must not eat a lot of heavy, greasy, rich food. One should also avoid uncooked, chilled, or hard food. . . . Of everything one eats and drinks, the most important thing is rice, which must be eaten in ample amounts to ensure proper nutrition. . . . Bean paste has a soft quality and is good for the stomach and intestines."[49]

Mizuno Namboku (1752-1825), Japan's greatest physiognomist, earned the reputation for telling at a glance everything about a person's health and destiny. But over the years, Mizuno discovered that some people's faces lied. They were able to defy the signs of illness, misfortune, and premature death engraved on their features. As he explains in *Food Governs Your Destiny*, which Aveline Kushi translated into English, dietary practice could alter one's fate. In an era in which food quality was completely organic and natural, controlling the quantity of food you ate, Mizuno explained, was more important than what you ate. In his own case, he ate primarily a small volume of barley (his main staple), soybeans, and other coarse foods. Mizuno eventually renounced the diagnostic arts and focused entirely on teaching about dietary practice and cultivating traditional virtues such as hard work, perseverance, patience, modesty, and concealing one's merits.[50]

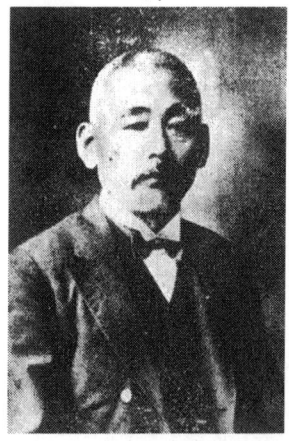

Sagen Ishizuka, M.D., a 19th century Japanese physician known as Dr. Miso Soup and Dr. Daikon

At the end of the 19th century, Japanese physician Sagen Ishizuka, M.D. (1850-1910) published the results of many years' research and study, outlining a broad theory of human physiology, food, health, sickness and medicine based on the dynamic balance between sodium and potassium in the environment and diet. On the basis of his own work as a military doctor in China and general practitioner in Japan, as well as readings in anthropology, he concluded that whole cereal grains contained the ideal balance of nutrients and should form the foundation of the human diet, supplemented with beans, vegetables, seeds and nuts, and a small amount of fish or game depending on the climate, region, and season of the year. In his clinic in Tokyo, he successfully treated many people with infectious diseases and was know as Dr. Miso Soup and Dr. Daikon because these were two foods he used in helping his patients recover.[51]

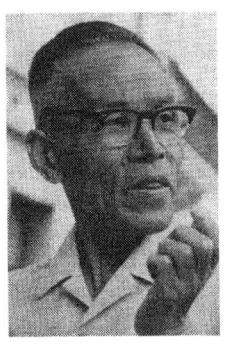

George Ohsawa, father of modern macrobiotics

Yukikazu Sakurazawa (1892-1966), a young man living in Kyoto, the old capital of Japan, cured himself of terminal tuberculosis in 1913 after reading a book on health and diet by Dr. Ishizuka. Over the next fifty years, under the penname George Ohsawa, he devoted his life to spreading a grain-based diet and guided thousands of people to health and happiness. He studied, traveled and taught in France, Belgium, and other parts of Europe in the 1920s and 1930s. During World War II, he was imprisoned for predicting that Japan would lose the war and for his peace activities. Liberated by the Americans at the end of the war, he set up a study house near Tokyo to promote a dietary approach to world peace under the name macrobiotics. Among his students were Michio Kushi and Tomoko Yokoyama, who went on to become leaders of the macrobiotic movement in America and internationally.

On a visit to Dr. Schweitzer's hospital in Central Africa in the 1950s with his wife Lima, Ohsawa hoped to impress the Nobel Prize winning physician with the benefits of macrobiotics. When Schweitzer ignored him, Ohsawa deliberately contracted tropical ulcers, a usually fatal tropical disease, and proceeded to heal himself with a macrobiotic regimen. In 1959, Ohsawa and Lima, came to the United States and gave the first formal macrobiotic lectures in New York City. He warned in early 1963 that President John F. Kennedy could be assassinated because of his *sanpaku* condition (extreme weakness shown by upturned eyes), and Tom Wolfe who attended his lecture proclaimed Ohsawa the new Nostradamus in the *New York Herald-Tribune*.[52] Ohsawa is widely considered the father of modern macrobiotics and wrote about 300 books and booklets, about a dozen of which are available in English.[53]

The philosophy of macrobiotics was succinctly expressed in the Statement of Purpose of the *East West Journal*, the Kushis' monthly magazine and voice of the counterculture in the 1970s and early 1980s. As editor Sherman Goldman wrote:

> *The East West Journal* explores the unity underlying apparently opposite values: Oriental and Occidental, traditional and modern, visionary and practical. We investigate the play of balance in all fields: from agriculture and nutrition through science and the arts, to politics and spirituality. We believe that people's freedom to chart the course of their lives as an endless adventure springs from the most basic factors of physical vitality. Our monthly how-to departments are inseparable from our feature articles on the frontiers of thought. We see humanity as a foreground figure set in a larger background of nature and the infinite universe. By creating our bodies and minds from whole foods in a spirit of thankfulness, we can recover our unity with the world, as parts in a common whole. We invite you to join us in this boundless

voyage of discovery. The compass we rely on in yin and yang; the staple fare we offer is macrobiotic; the dream toward which we steer is all humanity's.[54]

Dietary Practice

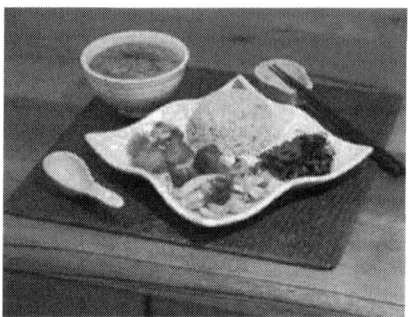

A typical macrobiotic meal consists of whole grains, miso soup, beans or bean products, vegetables from land and sea, pickles, tea, and fruit or a naturally sweetened dessert

The macrobiotic dietary approach has been practiced widely throughout history. Each culture and civilization has applied principles of balance to the proper selection and preparation of food and developed a unique cuisine in harmony with its natural environment. As Michio Kushi explained, "The macrobiotic approach is based not only on meeting optimal nutritional needs, but also on a deep understanding of the earth's relation to the sun, moon, and other celestial bodies; the evolution of life on the planet; ancestral tradition and heritage; ever-changing environmental and climatic conditions; humidity, pressure, and other atmospheric influences; local availability, affordability, and other economic factors; natural storability and other practical considerations; and the effects of different foods and beverages on mind, body, and spirit. The macrobiotic way of eating is not a set diet that applies rigidly to everyone, but a flexible dietary approach that differs according to climate, environment, condition of health, sex, age, activity level, and personal need."[55]

In the 2013 edition of *The Book of Macrobiotics*, Kushi introduced dietary guidelines for ten regions of the world, including Temperate Regions (such as North America, Europe, Russia, China, and Japan), Central America, South America, the Mediterranean, Middle East, Africa, South Asia, Southeast Asia and the Pacific Islands, a Cool Climate (Canada, Scotland, Scandinavia, Siberia), and a Cold Climate (Arctic). For each, he recommended varying amounts of grain, beans, vegetables fruits, and animal products depending on climate and environment.

Standard Macrobiotic Dietary Guidelines

In the United States, Michio and Aveline Kushi developed the Standard Macrobiotic Diet. Based on traditional cuisines and modern food patterns, daily meals in the temperate latitudes of the world ideally reflect the following categories and proportions of food:[56]

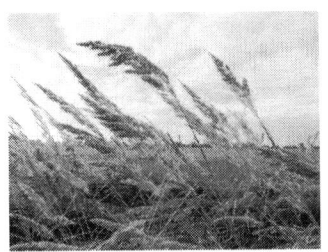

- **Whole Grains and Grain Products** 40 to 60 percent or more of daily food, by volume, consists of whole cereal grains and their products, representing the most advanced species of vegetable life. These include brown rice, whole wheat, barley, oats, rye, millet, corn, buckwheat, sorghum, and other traditional consumed wild and domesticated grasses
- **Soup** 5 to 10 percent of daily food may be taken in the form of soup (one to two bowls). The soup broth is made frequently with miso or shoyu, which are prepared from naturally fermented soybeans, sea salt, and grains, to which several varieties of land and sea vegetables may be added during cooking. The enzymes in miso and shoyu represent the most primordial form of life
- **Vegetables** 25 to 30 percent vegetables prepared in various ways, representing modern, ancient, and primordial stages of vegetal life. These include daikon, carrots, cabbage, kale, watercress, squashes, onion, and many other modern varieties; lotus root and other ancient species; and mushrooms and other primitive species
- **Beans and Sea Vegetables** 5 to 10 percent beans and bean products and sea vegetables representing more recent vegetable species from land and sea. These include azuki beans, chickpeas, lentils, pinto beans, soybeans and many others, as well as tofu, tempeh, and natto. Seaweeds and mosses include wakame, kombu, hijiki, nori, dulse, Irish moss, agar-agar, arame, and many others
- **Animal Food** Optional occasional use (15 percent or less) of animal food if desired, primarily fish and seafood, representing early animal life. These include cod, sole, trout, flounder, oyster, clam, shrimp, crab, and others
- **Fruits, Seeds, and Nuts** Occasional use of fruit, nuts, and seeds in small volume, representing the most recent biological species prior to grains. These include apples, cherries, peaches, plums, apricots, berries, melons, almonds, walnuts, pecans, cashews, sesame seeds, sunflower seeds, and pumpkin seeds, and many others
- **Fermented Food** Cultured food, especially that of vegetable quality, in small volume daily, representing the most primordial stage of biological life and strengthens the microbiome. Foods in this category containing beneficial enzymes and bacteria include miso, shoyu, koji (molded grain), natto, sauerkraut and other pickles, and many others
- **Seasonings and Condiments** White sea salt, shoyu (natural soy sauce), miso, umeboshi plums, unsaturated plant oils (especially sesame, olive, and safflower), rice vinegar, lemon, lime, and other citrus, and other traditionally used seasonings are used in cooking or at the table

- **Beverages** Daily beverages include kukicha tea (also known as bancha twig tea), roasted brown rice tea, roasted barley tea, and spring or well water. For occasional consumption, green tea, grain coffee, kombu tea, carrot or other vegetable juice, fruit juice, and other non-aromatic and non-stimulant drinks may be consumed. Beer, wine, or sake may taken for enjoyment on special occasions
- **Organic** Food to be organically grown as much as possible
- **Fire Quality** Cooking flame to be from gas, wood, charcoal, solar, or other natural source

Kitchenware

Cooking utensils should be made from natural and durable materials as much as possible such as wood, bamboo, glass, stainless steel and cast-iron while some materials including plastic, aluminum, copper, and non-stick coatings that may leach into food are to be avoided. A natural flame from gas, wood, charcoal, solar, or other natural source that gives a slow, steady source of energy is recommended while electric ovens and microwaves create a weaker, more chaotic vibration in the food should be avoided or minimized.[57]

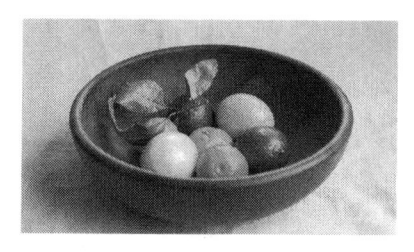

Wooden bowls and utensils give a natural energy and vibration

Lifestyle Guidelines

Macrobiotics promotes living in harmony with nature and striving for harmony and balance in all domains of life. The three pillars of health are 1) daily diet, 2) proper exercise or physical activity, and 3) intellectual or artistic pursuits, self-reflection, or spiritual practice. Standard way of life suggestions include:

- **Live Happily and Keep Active** Live each day happily without being preoccupied with your health. Try to keep mentally and physically active.
- **Be Grateful** View everything and everyone you meet with gratitude, particularly offering thanks before and after every meal
- **Early to Bed, Early to Rise** It is best to get up early and go to bed before midnight
- **Wear Natural Fabrics** It is best to wear cotton and other natural fiber clothing, especially for undergarments, and to use cotton bed sheets and pillows. Avoid GMO cotton and synthetic or woolen clothing directly on the skin and avoid excessive metallic accessories on the fingers, wrists, or neck. Keep such ornaments simple and graceful

- **Go Outside and Keep Home in Order** If your strength permits, go outdoors in simple clothing. Walk on the grass, beach, or soil up to one half hour each day. Keep your home in good order, from the kitchen, bathroom, bedroom, and living room, to every corner
- **Keep in Touch** Initiate and maintain an active correspondence, extending best wishes to parents, children, brothers and sisters, and friends by ordinary mail, email, texting, Skype, or phone
- **Avoid Long Bathing** Avoid taking long, hot baths or showers unless you have been consuming too much salt or animal food, as these take minerals from the body
- **Be Active** If your condition permits, exercise regularly as part of daily life, including activities like walking, scrubbing floors, cleaning windows, washing clothes, and working in the garden. You may also engage in exercise programs such as yoga, martial arts, dance, or sports
- **Minimize Electronics** Minimize the frequent use of television, computers, cell phones, and other electronics that emit artificial electromagnetic radiation
- **Oxygenate Your Home with Green Plants** Include some large green plants in your house to freshen and enrich the oxygen content of the air of your home
- **Be Kind to Animals** Treat animals, birds, insects, and all living things respectively
- **Sing a Happy Song** Sing a happy song every day

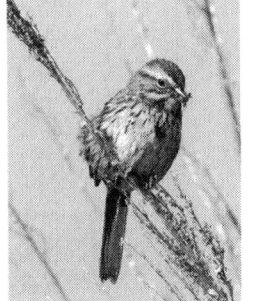

Learn from nature.
Sing a happy song
each day

Progressive Development of Disease

In contrast to modern medicine that classifies disease into hundreds of categories, macrobiotic healthcare looks at sickness as a progressive pattern of seven stages:

1. General Fatigue: Physical tiredness, often accompanied by muscular tension and a hardening of the muscles, frequent urination and sweating, temporary constipation or diarrhea, and short periods of feeling cold or hot. Mentally we start to lose our clarity of thought, active perception and accurate responses. To recover from this stage, it usually takes a short period—from a few hours to a few days—of adequate rest, a good night's sleep, proper food and drink, and exercise.

2. Aches and Pains: When a feeling of general fatigue prevails, occasional pains and aches may develop. Muscular pain, headache, cramps, and various other sorts of pains and aches appear now and then. Temporary shortness of breath, irregular heartbeat, fever and chills, and difficulty of motion also appear in this stage. Mentally, we may experience occasional depression, worry, and a general feeling of insecurity. To restore health usually takes from a few days to a few weeks, with proper dietary practice, active exercise, or necessary rest.

3. Blood Disease: If our dietary practice continues to be out of balance with our environment, our blood quality, including red blood cells, white blood cells, and blood plasma, becomes unsuited for maintaining harmony with our natural surroundings. The quality of our blood determines the quality of our body's cells and tissues, organs, and systems. Blood disorders create various abnormal conditions in our body from which symptoms of sickness then arise. Acidosis (a condition in which there is too much acid in the body fluids), high and low blood pressure, anemia, purpura (purple-colored spots and patches that occur on the skin caused by bleeding from small blood vessels under the skin), leukemia, scurvy, and other diseases belong to this stage, including asthma, epilepsy, and skin diseases. Mentally, this stage appears as nervousness, hypersensitivity, complaining, pessimism, timidity, and loss of general direction in life. To recover from blood disorders may take between 10 days and three to four months, depending upon the individual condition. Once again, proper dietary practices, as well as suitable exercise and rest, need to be implemented. Simple home cares to promote active circulation of the blood may also be required in some cases.

4. Emotional Disorder: If an improper quality of blood circulates for a prolonged period, various emotional disorders start to appear. Short temper, excitement, anger, frustration, melancholy, and a general feeling of despair are experienced frequently in daily life. A gentle approach to a problem with clear, balanced understanding is no longer possible. A general feeling of fear prevails toward new situations and surroundings, and our daily behavior and way of thinking become extremely defensive or offensive. Our physical movements become more rigid, and we gradually lose flexibility in both body and mind. It requires between one month and several months to overcome these emotional and physical disorders. Dietary change toward more balanced food is essential, along with physical and mental relaxation.

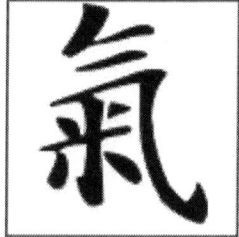

The ideogram for Ki, or life energy, is the steam rising from cooked rice. Illness is known in the East as "bad Ki" often arising from poor food choices

5. Organ Disease An imbalanced quality of blood circulating for a prolonged period further produces gradual changes in the quality and function of our organs and glands. Structural change, malfunction, and degeneration start to arise. Atherosclerosis (a hardening of the arteries), diabetes, stone formation in the kidneys or gallbladder, arthritis, various types of cancer, diabetes, various types of cancer, and many other chronic diseasesfall in this category. Mentally, chronic stubbornness, prejudice, narrow-mindedness, and general rigidity with a distorted view of life become more apparent. To recover from this level of disease usually takes several months to one year or more, through continuous practice of proper diet and reorientation of the way of life, including deep self-reflection.

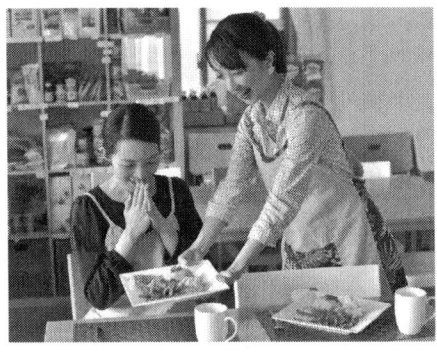

Gratitude is the key to overcoming many difficulties and illnesses

6. Nervous Disorder: From the stage of organ and gland disease, the degenerative tendency progresses toward various nervous disorders including physical paralysis, Alzheimer's disease, and mental illness including bipolar disease, schizophrenia, and paranoia. Physical and mental coordination of various functions gradually diminishes. A negative view begins to dominate daily life, and suicidal or destructive tendencies frequently manifest. It takes six months to a few years to recover completely from this stage and to regain self-assurance and trust as well as a positive view of life. The way of life has to be changed completely, including dietary practice, more harmonious relationship with the environment, and active physical exercise, together with loving care by family and friends.

7. Self-Centeredness An improper way of life that has been practiced for many years, finally reaches the highest level of sickness—self-centeredness or arrogance—though some of the previous stages may not have been clearly experienced. Self-centeredness is the most developed sickness and also the one that most universally affects people's lives today. Selfishness, egocentricity, vanity, self-pride, exclusivity, and self-justification are some of the common symptoms. It is the last stage of sickness and, at the same time, it is the cause of all previous stages. To overcome this attitude takes from a few years to an indefinite length of time of proper practice in a more appreciative and natural way of life. However, it can also be cured instantaneously through strong emotional or spiritual experiences, especially in the face of great difficulties and failure. The cure of self-centeredness immediately produces a spirit of humility and modesty. It restores also the spirit of appreciation through the recognition of our ignorance. When arrogance is dissolved, a new way of life in harmony with the environment automatically begins.

As Michio Kushi observed, "Every physical, mental, and spiritual sickness belongs to one of the seven levels outlined above, though symptoms at some of the steps may remain dormant and unrecognized. All sicknesses are interdependent and interconnected with one another; they are symptoms branching out from the same root—improper way of life. As long as we follow and live according to the laws of nature and the Order of the Universe, as our ancestors have done from the beginning, we shall enjoy health, happiness, and longevity, rarely suffering from any form of sickness."[58]

Natural Healing

From the "macro" or largest view, macrobiotics embraces all the diverse traditions and products of human culture and tradition, including modern medicine and new nutritional and energetic techniques. The Mandala of Healing, created by Michio Kushi, illustrates the seven levels of healing (*mandala* = Sanskrit for wheel or spiral):

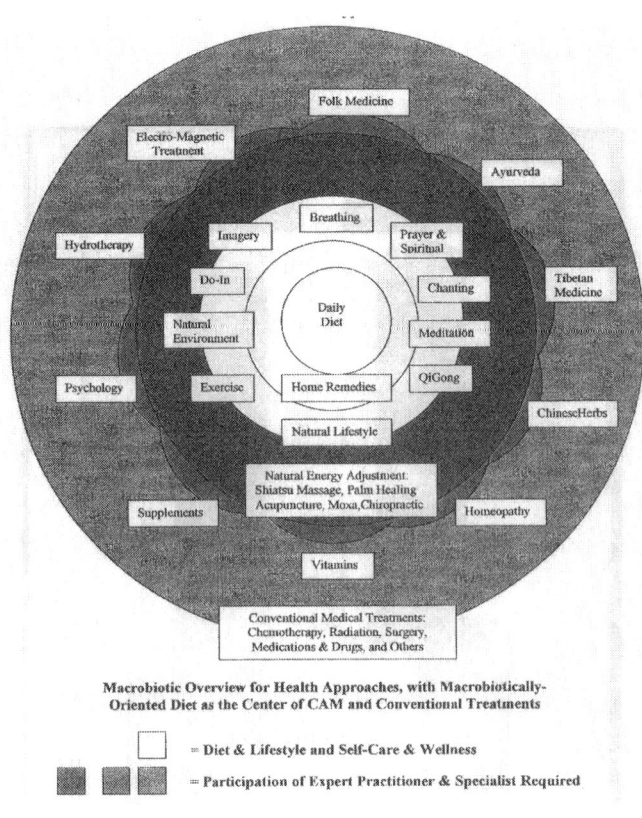

Macrobiotic Overview for Health Approaches, with Macrobiotically-Oriented Diet as the Center of CAM and Conventional Treatments

☐ = Diet & Lifestyle and Self-Care & Wellness

■ ■ ■ = Participation of Expert Practitioner & Specialist Required

1. Daily Way of Eating. At the center of the mandala of healing is dietary practice, namely, the macrobiotic way of eating. This approach itself is constantly evolving to take into account changing environmental and climactic conditions, social and economic factors, and personal needs. It comprises the foundation of healing.

2. Home Remedies: In principle, a balanced daily way of eating will help prevent sickness and harm. But if imbalance arises, special dishes, special drinks, and home remedies (most of which are based on traditional foods such as the ginger compress, ume-sho-kuzu drink, and cabbage leaf plaster) represent the next, or second circle of healing.

3. Natural Lifestyle: The third circle represents natural lifestyle approaches and includes simple activities and exercises that can be used to strengthen mind and body, stimulate energy flow, and promote better metabolism at various levels. Examples: do-in, or self-massage, yoga, tai chi and qi gong, walking, painting and drawing, dance, singing, playing or listening to music, prayer, meditation, mind control, and other simple, basic practices that can be performed by oneself easily, safely, and without any special cost.

4. Natural Energy Adjustments: The fourth level of healing involves natural energy adjustments. Examples include acupuncture (the use of needles to stimulate energy flow), moxibustion (the use of a dried herb for similar purposes), shiatsu or massage that makes use of clay or oils, aromatherapy, chiropractic, osteopathy, neurolinguistic programming, and others. Again, these external applications may be helpful depending on the case, but they generally require a second person to administer, usually an expert, and involve specialized diagnosis and evaluation, and entail an expense. Compared to the first three circles, level four represents moving beyond self-reliance to dependence on authorities, companies, and health claims that may or may not be true and beneficial.

5. Supplements and Special Products. The fifth circle of healing includes supplements, vitamins, minerals, herbs, and other largely nutritional products. They include both traditional substances such as Chinese herbs and modern extracts such as genistein (soy-based) tablets and homeopathic tinctures. For the most part, they originate from natural plants or animals, but the way they are processed may be calm and peaceful (like macrobiotic cooking) or highly processed (like fast foods). They may also contain other ingredients of low quality (such as gelatin, or animal-based, capsules), and they can be rather expensive and in some cases require an expert to prescribe or administer.

6. Electromagnetic Treatments. The sixth circle includes electric, radionic, digital, and other electromagnetic gadgets, devices, and machines. Again, these external applications may be helpful for any given person, but they may not be suitable for others and are often invasive, require experts, and incur significant cost.

7. Conventional Medicine. The seventh circle includes conventional medical procedures. The most innocuous are blood tests, EKGs, and other simple lab tests. A variety of pills, drugs, and medications carry moderate to high risks, especially SSRI's and other psychiatric drugs. Other risky procedures include surgery (which may range from mild to life-threatening but which can damage meridian flow), radiation of different kinds (MRIs, CT scans, X-rays, mammograms), chemotherapy, and many experimental medications. Except for accidents, emergencies, and life-and-death situations, many medical procedures are unnecessary, aimed at destroying disease rather than identifying the underlying cause of imbalance. However, in any given case, they may be beneficial (especially temporarily and in small, controlled amounts or frequencies), necessary, or lifesaving.

The mandala encourages us to develop our intuition, starting at the center and taking as much responsibility as we can for our own health and well-being. However, it prompts us to use wider, more complex methods and procedures as necessary. It is common sense to keep an open mind to all manner of healing but also to use the invasive, risky, and costly ones as a last, rather than a first, resort.

Scientific and Medical Studies

Ancient Nutrition
The opening story in the Book of Daniel in the Bible is the world's oldest nutrition experiment.

⚕ The Book of Daniel

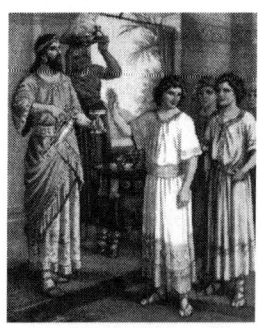

Young Daniel requests a simple, grain-based diet at the palace of the King of Babylon

During the Babylonian Captivity, King Nebuchadnezzar commanded several of the most gifted young men of Israel to be brought to court to enter the royal service. The king instructed Malasar, the master of his household, to feed Daniel and his three companions the best meat and wine from the royal table. The Israelites, however, refused the rich food and instead asked for the simple meals they were accustomed to. The steward rejected their request, fearing that he would lose his head if the king saw Daniel and his friends undernourished in comparison to the young Babylonians their age also in training for royal service. Daniel replied: "Try, I beseech thee, thy servants for ten days, and let pulse [whole grains, lentils, seeds] be given us to eat, and water to drink. And look upon our faces, and the faces of the children that eat of the king's meat: and as thou shalt see, deal with thy servants. And when he had heard these words, he tried them for ten days. And after ten days their faces appeared fairer and fatter than all the children that ate of the king's meat. So Malasar took their portions, and the wine that they should drink: and he gave them pulse. And to these children God gave knowledge and understanding in every book, and wisdom: but to Daniel the understanding also of all visions and dreams."[59]

As the world's first nutrition experiment, the episode involves two groups (an intervention group of young Jews and a control group of young Babylonians), dietary variables (a plant vs. animal-based diet), a set duration (10 days), observable outcomes (change in countenance, disposition, and physique), and an impartial investigator (steward of the palace of the king of Babylon). As a result of his macrobiotic diet and divine favor, Daniel became the principal adviser to the King, a great prophet, and leader who helped deliver his people from captivity.

Macrobiotic Nutrition

In comparison with the standard modern way of eating, the macrobiotic dietary approach has the following general nutritional characteristics:[60]

- **More Complex Carbohydrates** Fewer simple sugars and more complex carbohydrates
- **More Plant Protein** More vegetable-quality protein, less animal quality protein
- **Less Fat and Oil** Less overall fat consumption, more polyunsaturated fat, and less saturated fat
- **Less Supplements** A balance of various naturally occurring vitamins, minerals and other nutrients and less supplementation
- **More Organic Food** Use of more organically grown, natural food and more traditional food processing techniques and less chemically grown, artificially produced, or chemically processed foods
- **More Whole Food** Consumption of food primarily in whole form and less refined, partial, or processed food
- **More Natural Food** Greater consumption of food that is high in natural fiber, antioxidants, and phytoestrogens and less food that has been devitalized by overprocessing, genetic engineering, irradiation, or other artificial technologies

Over the years, scientific and medical studies have generally found that the macrobiotic way of eating meets current nutritional guidelines. These studies include:

⚕ Landmark Report Links Diet with Degenerative Disease

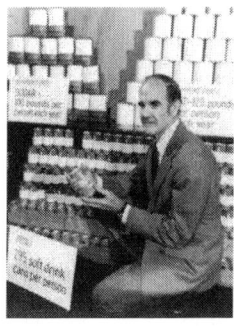

Senator George McGovern shows the harmful effects of sugar and soft drinks on public health

Summarizing its conclusions on the nation's way of eating, health, and future direction, the historic Senate report, *Dietary Goals for the United States* (also known as the McGovern Report after its chairman, former Democratic presidential candidate George McGovern) launched the modern nutritional revolution in 1977: "During this century, the composition of the average diet in the United States has changed radically. Complex carbohydrates— fruit, vegetables, and grain products—which were the mainstay of the diet, now play a minority role. At the same time, fat and sugar consumption have risen to the point where these two dietary elements alone now comprise at least 60 percent of total calorie intake, up from 50 percent in the early 1900s. In the view of doctors and nutritionists consulted by the Select Committee, these and other changes in the diet amount to a wave of malnutrition—of both over- and underconsumption—that may be as profoundly damaging to the Nation's health as the widespread contagious diseases of the early part of this century. The overconsumption of fat, generally, and saturated fat in particular, as well as cholesterol, sugar, salt, and alcohol have been related to six of the leading causes of death: Heart disease, cancer, cerebrovascular diseases, diabetes, arteriosclerosis, and cirrhosis of the liver."

Macrobiotic educators Michio and Aveline Kushi; the East West Foundation under the leadership of Edward Esko and Stephen Uprichard; and *East West Journal* under Sherman Goldman, Alex Jack, and Tom Monte wrote about the relationship of diet and degenerative disease and prepared materials or met with key experts and witnesses in the hearings.[61]

⚕ Macrobiotic Practice Meets Nutritional Guidelines

Researchers at the University of Rhode Island studied 76 macrobiotic people and reported in the *Journal of the American Dietetic Association* in 1980 they met currently acceptable medical and nutritional guidelines, including mean values for hemoglobin, hematocrit, serum iron, and transferrin saturation, serum ascorbic acid, vitamin A, beta-carotene, riboflavin, vitamin B-12, and folate.[62]

⚕ Macrobiotic Diet Meets or Exceeds British RDAs

At the University of London, researchers measured the dietary intakes of 10 people practicing macrobiotics and they were found to be adequate in all major nutrients of the United Kingdom Recommended Daily amounts. All of the other nutrients either met the RDA's or, in the case of vitamins A and C, thiamine, calcium, and iron, "far exceeded the recommendations." "The macrobiotic diet as eaten by the participants of this study was found to conform with many of the recommendations put forward by recent [medical and scientific] reports on eating for health," according to the chief researcher's report in 1985.[63]

⚕ The China Study

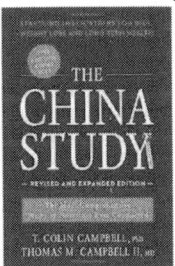

The world's most comprehensive nutrition study supports a macrobiotic way of eating. A Chinese research project, hailed as the "Grand Prix of Epidemiology," challenged modern dietary assumptions. Sponsored by the U.S. National Cancer Institute and the Chinese Institute of Nutrition and Food Hygiene, the decade-long study in the 1990s correlated average food and nutrient intakes with disease mortality rates in 65 rural Chinese counties. The typical Chinese diet included a high proportion of cereal grains and vegetables and a low content of animal food. Less than 1 percent of deaths were caused by coronary heart disease, cancer, and other chronic diseases common in the West.

Study director Dr. T. Colin Campbell, a professor of nutrition at Cornell University and member of the expert committee that developed the U.S. Food Guide Pyramid, concluded:

- **Reduce Fat** Fat consumption should ideally be reduced to 10 to 15 percent of calories to prevent degenerative disease, not 30 percent as usually recommended
- **Eat More Plant-Based Foods** The lowest risk for cancer is generated by the consumption of a variety of fresh plant products
- **Reduce Animal Protein** Eating animal protein is a main cause of chronic disease. Compared to the Chinese who derive 11 percent of their protein from animal sources, Americans obtain 70 percent from animal food
- **Natural Menstruation** A rich diet that promotes early menstruation may increase a woman's risk of cancer of the breast and reproductive organs. In the West, girls typically begin to menstruate at 11, in China at 17
- **Strengthen Bones by Avoiding Dairy** Dairy food is not needed to prevent osteoporosis, the thinning of the bones that is common

among older women, and indeed may be a cause for bone loss

- **Eat Leafy Greens for Iron** Meat consumption is not needed to prevent iron-deficiency anemia. The average Chinese consumes twice the iron Americans do, primarily from plant sources, and show no signs of anemia

Dr. Campbell, who grew up on a dairy farm, because a vegan as a result of his studies and frequently lectures at macrobiotic conferences. The healthy traditional Chinese diet, he explains, is essentially macrobiotic.[64]

Higher in Iron and Other Nutrients Than Standard Diet

Researchers at the University of Memphis and University of South Carolina evaluated the dietary pattern at the Kushi Institute's Way to Health program and concluded in a 2015 article in *Nutrition and Cancer* that it had a lower percentage of potentially harmful fats, higher total dietary fiber, and higher amounts of most micronutrients, including beta-carotene, B vitamins, and iron, than the standard American diet. "Findings from this analysis of a macrobiotic diet plan indicate the potential for disease prevention and suggest the need for studies of real-world consumption as well as designing, implementing, and testing interventions based on the macrobiotic approach," the scientists concluded.[65]

Rich in Nutrient-Dense Foods

In an article on the popular website WebMD.com, Dr. Michael Smith observed in 2016: "If you're looking for a healthy eating plan, the macrobiotic diet is a good choice. It's rich in nutrient-packed foods that are also low in calories. While there's no absolute proof, medical research suggests diets that are mostly vegetables, fruits, and whole grains may lower the risk of several diseases, including heart disease and cancer. Either way, you'll reap plenty of health benefits with this diet."[66]

Heart Disease

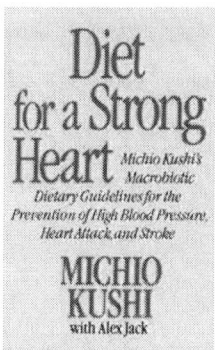

In the early 1970s, Frank Sachs, a student at Harvard Medical School, was impressed with Michio Kushi's lectures and arranged with his professors at Channing Laboratory to begin the first medical studies on macrobiotics. They focused on blood pressure, cholesterol levels, and other basic blood values. Several hundred members of the macrobiotic community volunteered for what turned out to be a series of studies that were published in the *New England Journal of Medicine*, *Atheroclerosis*, and other major journals. The studies convincingly linked diet and heart disease, which until then had been largely neglected, and led to the first national dietary guidelines on the number one cause of death in modern society. The macrobiotic approach, including these studies, was featured in Michio Kushi's *Diet for a Strong Heart*.

⚕ Boston Macrobiotics at Zero Risk for Heart Disease

In a study of 210 men and women eating a macrobiotic diet, Harvard Medical School researchers found that the men had mean systolic blood pressures of 109.7 mm Hg and diastolic pressures of 60.9. The women had 100.9 and 58.2 respectively. Both of these measurements fell well within the normal blood pressure category and approached the systolic level of 100 under which Framingham Heart Study researchers theorized there would develop virtually no coronary heart disease.[67]

⚕ Average Macrobiotic Cholesterol 126

Harvard Medical School researchers reported that Boston-area macrobiotic people had significantly lower cholesterol and triglyceride levels and lower blood pressure than a control group from the Framingham Heart Study eating the standard American diet of meat, sugar, dairy foods, and highly processed, chemicalized foods. The average serum cholesterol in the macrobiotic group was 126 milligrams per deciliter versus 184 for controls. "The low plasma lipid levels in the vegetarians," the researchers concluded in the *New England Journal of Medicine*, "resemble those reported for populations in nonindustrialized societies" where heart disease, cancer, and other degenerative illnesses are uncommon.[68]

⚕ Surgeon General Cites Macrobiotic Diet for Heart Health

In his annual report in 1979, the U.S. Surgeon General reported for the first time that existing coronary heart disease could be relieved by dietary measures. "Direct evidence from animal studies supports the linkage of atherosclerosis with high levels of fats (particularly saturated) and cholesterol in the diet . . . [and] that Americans who habitually eat less fat rich foods ([macrobiotic] vegetarians and Seventh Day Adventists, for example) have less heart disease than other Americans; and that atherosclerotic plaques in certain arteries may be reversed by cholesterol-lowering diets."[69]

⚕ Pioneer Study Links Animal Food and High Blood Pressure

In one of the first studies to show the direct effects of animal food on raising blood pressure, a study of 21 macrobiotic persons by Harvard Medical School researchers in 1981 found that the addition of 250 grams of beef per day for four weeks to their regular diet of whole grains and vegetables raised serum cholesterol levels 19 percent. Systolic blood pressure also rose significantly. After returning to a low-fat diet, cholesterol and blood pressure values returned to previous levels, the researchers reported in *the Journal of the American Medical Association*).[70]

☤ Macrobiotic Practitioners Healthier Than Marathon Runners

William Castelli, M.D., director of the Framingham Heart Study, the nation's oldest and largest cardiovascular research project, and a participant in research on macrobiotic people at Harvard Medical School, noted that macrobiotic people have healthier hearts and circulatory systems than conditioned athletes: "What a person eats every day is a very important aspect of how his or her health will be in every day as well as later life. Supporting this view is the fact that macrobiotic people studied had a ratio [of total cholesterol to HDL cholesterol of] 2.5 and Boston marathon runners were at 3.4, ratios at which rarely, if ever, is coronary heart disease seen. Studies and observations such as these are a clear indicator that people need to take a critical look at their diet with the intention of making changes now."[71]

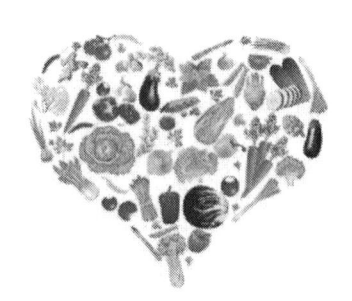

☤ Macrobiotics Aids Angina Patients in New York Hospital

Physicians at Columbia Presbyterian Hospital in New York City reported that patients with angina pectoris, showed improved blood pressure values and lowered coronary risk factors after ten weeks on a macrobiotic diet and treatment with biofeedback. Dr. Kenneth Greenspan of the hospital's Laboratory and Center for Stress Related Disorders, reported that cholesterol dropped from an average 300 to 220, levels of blood pressure also dropped, patients could walk about 20 percent farther in stress tests, and three patients with severe angina showed no symptoms at the end of the study.[72]

Cancer

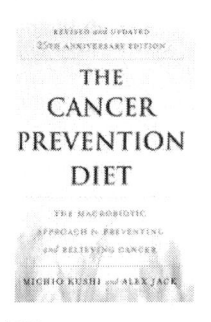

During the 20th century, the incidence of cancer in modern society soared, rising from 2% of the population in 1900 to 25% in the 1950s and 1960s. There was no effective treatment or cure, and many people felt it marked a death sentence. In Boston, Michio Kushi began to give personal dietary and way of life consultations, and many cancer patients came to him for advice. The first person to experience complete remission following a macrobiotic way of eating was Professor Jean Kohler, a university instructor in music at Ball State College in Indiana, who had pancreatic cancer, a nearly always fatal illness. Following his successful recovery in the late 1970s, the Kushis and their associates began to focus on cancer, especially now that the medical studies at Harvard and the Framingham Heart Study had shown that a balanced, whole foods diet could bring down high blood pressure, lower cholesterol, and reduce the risk of heart disease.[73]

The *East West Journal*, the macrobiotic monthly magazine, focused on cancer and diet, publishing macrobiotic case histories, and investigating the ties of the medical profession to the food industry. Journalist Peter Barry Chowka wrote several influential investigative articles on the American Cancer Society and National Cancer Institute and their neglect of dietary and lifestyle factors in the etiology of the disease. The East West Foundation, under the Kushis's auspices, sponsored the first Conference on Cancer and Diet, at Pine Manor College in Brookline, MA in 1977. The gathering brought together physicians, researchers, and many patients who had recovered using a macrobiotic approach. St. Martin's Press brought out Kushi's major book, *The Cancer-Prevention Diet*, co-authored by Alex Jack, editor-in-chief of *East West Journal,* in 1983. The book was translated into more than a dozen languages and included chapters on 20 major types of cancer, including a description of the food patterns underling their cause, dietary guidelines for recovery, home remedies, and lifestyle suggestions.

Over the years, hundreds—possibly thousands—of people, recovered from cancer with the help of macrobiotics. At the Kushi Institute in Becket, Massachusetts, the main residential center for macrobiotic education, the one-week Way to Health Program introduced individuals and families, many with cancer or other chronic diseases, to the principles and practices of macrobiotics, including daily cooking classes, menu planning, and proper use of home remedies. Many people who met with Michio Kushi or other counselors, or who attended programs at the K.I. (or affiliated campuses around the world) went on to lead healthy, fulfilling lives and chronicled their healing stories in their own books or articles. These included:

- **Businessman Heals Pancreatic Cancer** Norman Arnold, a businessman from South Carolina, who recovered from pancreatic cancer. He went on to live cancer-free for another 35 years and establish the Cancer Center at the University of South Carolina that employed several macrobiotic-oriented researchers.[74]
- **Journalist Heals Metastatic Ovarian and Lymph Cancer** Milenka Dobic, a journalist from Yugoslavia with ovarian and lymph cancer. She went on to become a leading macrobiotic teacher and counselor and described her recovery in *My Beautiful Life*.[75]

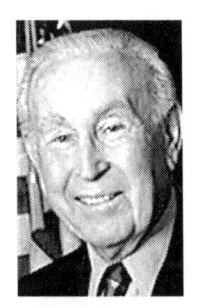

Norman Arnold recovered from pancreatic cancer

- **Hollywood Star Recovers from Prostate Cancer** Dirk Benedict, the actor and star of *The A-Team* and *Battlestar Galactica*, who recovered from prostate cancer.[76]
- **Mother Overcomes Inoperable Uterine Tumor** Elaine Nussbaum, a mother from New Jersey with an inoperable uterine tumor, who went on to become a leading macrobiotic teacher and cook.[77]
- **United Nations Official Recovers from Stomach Cancer** Katsuhide Kitatani, deputy Secretary-General of the United Nations, who had stomach cancer. He went on to found the U.N. Macrobiotic Society and 2050, a nonprofit development organization in Southeast Asia.[78]
- **Brain Tumor Overcome** Mona Sanders, a young woman from Columbus, Mississippi, had a brain tumor. After recovering, she served as an assistant to Michio Kushi and moved to India, where she taught diet and health for the next 25 years.[79]
- **Physician and Hospital President Heals Prostate Cancer** Anthony Sattilaro, M.D., president of Methodist Hospital in Philadelphia, who had metastatic prostate cancer that spread to the bones, testicles, and other internal organs. Within a few weeks of starting a macrobiotic diet, the back pain he suffered for years eased, and after several months his tumors went away. One-year and four-year follow up scans at his own hospital confirmed that the cancer had completely disappeared. Dr. Sattilaro was profiled in *East West Journal, Saturday Evening Post* and *Life* magazines and went on to write a bestselling book with Tom Monte *Recalled By Life*.[80]
- **Nurse Overcomes Metastatic Lung Cancer** Janet E. Vitt, R.N., a nurse in Cleveland, had stage 4 lung cancer that had spread to her liver, pancreas, abdomen, and lymph system. After exhausting her medical options, she went to a macrobiotic counselor and after 10 months the tumors were all gone. Jane went on to become a macrobiotic cook, teacher, and counselor, guiding many people to greater health and well-being.[81]
- **Nurse Reverses Malignant Melanoma** Virginia Brown, R.N., a nurse in Vermont, recovered from malignant melanoma. Her story appeared in *Macrobiotic Miracle*.[82]
- **Physician Documents Husband's Recovery from Colon Cancer** Vivian Newbold, M.D., a Philadelphia physician chronicled the recovery of her husband who had colon cancer.[83]

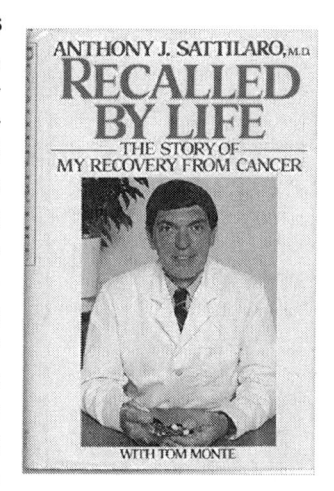

Leukemia Survivor Turned Celebrity Chef Christina Pirello, a young woman with leukemia, married her macrobiotic counselor, Bob Pirello, and went on to become a macrobiotic teacher, chef, and Emmy-award winning star of the longtime PBS-TV show *Christina Cooks!*[84]

Businessman Heals Prostate Cancer Ken Walles, a Long Island businessman, healed himself of prostate cancer with the help of macrobiotics. Through the Oceanside Beach Resort in Montauk, NY he observes a healthy diet and lifestyle.[85]

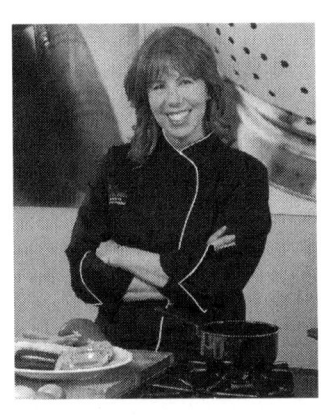

After healing herself of leukemia, Christina Pirello became host of PBS's *Christina Cooks*

Personal accounts are among the most powerful and convincing testimony on the benefits of macrobiotics. However, for the medical community, these claims needed to be evaluated scientifically. Over the years, there have been studies of the macrobiotic approach to cancer by the NIH, CDC, and other medical organizations and research centers:

NIH Best Case Series of 77 Macrobiotic Cancer Recoveries

The National Institute of Health's (NIH) Macrobiotic Best Case Series undertaken by researchers at the University of Minnesota in the 1990s, documented the medical histories of 77 individuals who recovered from cancer with the help of macrobiotics. These included cancers of the prostate (20 cases), breast (12 cases), malignant melanoma (8), lymphoma (8), leukemia (6), astrocytoma (5), colorectal (4), endometrium (3), ovary (3), pancreas (3), kidney (2), liver (1), small cell lung (1), multiple myeloma (1), nose plasmacytoma (1), parotic gland (1), sarcoma (1), and small intestine (1).[86]

NCI Approves Clinical Study on Macrobiotics and Cancer

The Cancer Advisory Panel on Complementary and Alternative Medicine (CAPCAM), an expert committee of oncologists from the National Institute of Cancer (NCI), in 2003 reviewed the cases of six persons who had been diagnosed with IVth stage metastasized cancer and were part of the NIH Best Cases Series. The review included viewing patient slides and records, hearing expert testimony from a radiologist and pathologist, and listening to an explanation on macrobiotic theory and practice by Michio Kushi. In addition, three of the six persons whose cases were being reviewed gave personal testimony and answered questions from the panelists. At the end of a day-long, rigorous review, the panel of 15 physicians and scientists voted unanimously to recommend to the NCI that governmental funding should be provided for a prospective and full clinical study on macrobiotics and cancer.[87]

⚕ CDC Reviews 51 Macrobiotic Healing Cases
In a study sponsored by the Centers for Disease Control and Disease Prevention (CDC), the public health arm of the United States, cancer researchers at the School of Public Health, University of South Carolina, investigated the macrobiotic way of life from 2000-2002. In a report "Macrobiotics in the United States: An Assessment of Services and Activities," Sheldon and Ginat Rice interviewed 124 practitioners in 44 locales. Fifty-one people recounted personal healing stories in which macrobiotic practice reversed a serious health condition. Of these, twenty-one were instances of cancer and four more were pre-cancerous cysts. The researchers posted a selection of recovery stories from cancer and other chronic diseases on the Internet along with a list of macrobiotic resources, including educational centers, teachers and counselors, and books and other study materials for the use of the general public.[88]

⚕ M.D. Anderson Cancer Center Reviews Macrobiotics
Cancer researchers at M.D. Anderson Cancer Center at the University of Texas in Houston posted a historical overview of macrobiotics as a therapy for cancer patients and the general public on their web site in early 2003. "The macrobiotic diet is part of a way of life that attempts to achieve balance by applying the oriental principles of yin and yang to the selection of foods. According to one study, 63% of cancer patients who received some form of dietary therapy received or were exposed to the macrobiotic diet."[89]

Breast Cancer
Breast cancer is the most common form of cancer in American women, and about 1 in 8 will contract this disease. Many women have recovered following a macrobiotic approach, and medical studies found that the diet leads to improved processing of estrogen and other hormones and improved microflora in the gut:

⚕ Macrobiotic Women Less Likely to Develop Breast Cancer
Macrobiotic and vegetarian women are less likely to develop breast cancer, researchers at New England Medical Center in Boston reported in 1981. The scientists found that macrobiotic and vegetarian women process estrogen differ-

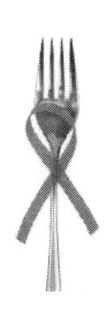

ently from other women and eliminate it more quickly from their body. "The difference in estrogen metabolism may explain the lower incidence of breast cancer in vegetarian [macrobiotic] women," the study published in *Cancer Research* concluded.[90]

☤ Kombu Protects Against Breast Cancer

Jane Teas, Ph.D., a researcher at Harvard University, and her colleagues found that kombu, a thick green seaweed that is a part of the regular macrobiotic way of eating, protected against breast cancer in laboratory studies.[91] In another study, a Japanese researcher reported that rats fed sea vegetables had about half the induced breast cancer rate than controls.[92]

☤ Macrobiotic Diet Reduces Tumor Risk in Italian Women

In a random case control study involving 104 middle-aged women at high risk for breast cancer, researchers at the National Tumor Institute in Milan, Italy, reported that a macrobiotic diet could substantially reduce hormonal levels associated with higher risk for this malignancy. The intervention group lost more weight, 4.06 kg compared to 0.54 kg, and underwent statistically significant improvements in the five major hormonal and metabolic values associated with breast cancer risk: sex hormone-binding globulin, testosterone, estradiol, fasting insulin, and fasting glycemia. Serum sex hormone-binding globulin levels increased 25.2%, while testosterone and estradiol decreased 19.5% and 18%. "We observed significant and favorable changes in hormonal indicators of breast cancer risk in a group of postmenopausal women living in northern Italy," the researchers concluded. "These results suggest that the multifactorial dietary intervention applied in this study may prevent breast cancer if continued in the long term." "Compared with the usual Western microflora, the gut of macrobiotic or vegetarian subjects may be richer in lactobacilli and bifidobacteria," the scientists noted in an article in *Cancer Epidemiology, Biomarkers, & Prevention*. The study led to a series of further studies on the effectiveness of the macrobiotic approach to this illness.[93]

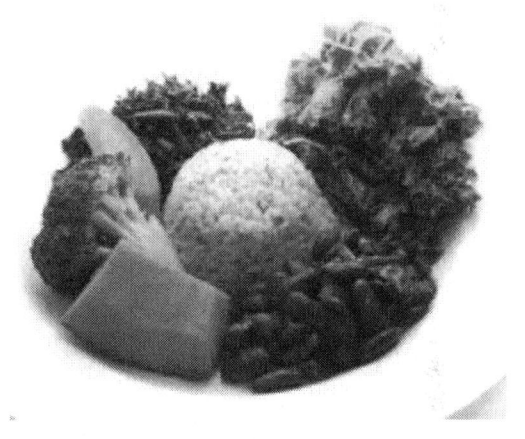

Breast cancer risk fell on a macrobiotic diet

☥ Diet Lowers Risk of BRCA Breast Cancer

A plant-based diet lowers the risk of breast cancer for women who test positive for BRCA. In a review of the medical literature, Alex Jack found that a plant-based diet resulted in lower IGF-1 levels (reducing risk up to 7 times or 85%) among women testing positive for the BRCA gene mutation.[94] Higher consumption of fruits and vegetables reduced risk between 72 and 82%.[95] Lower weight brought the risk down between 80 and 90%. Breastfeeding reduced risk by 45% (BRCA1 type only).[96] He concluded that the well-publicized case of Angelina Jolie who had a double mastectomy was especially tragic because she had already altered her diet and breastfed her children, bringing her risk down to normal. Her doctors told her without surgery she had an 87% higher risk of breast or ovarian cancer. Neither Jolie nor her doctors appear to have known of these studies.

About 1-2% of women of Scandinavian, Icelandic, Dutch, and Ashkenazi Jewish heritage carry the BRCA mutation. Jack hypothesized that the BRCA, a normal DNA repair gene, mutated several centuries ago when dairy food consumption in these regions increased as society became more affluent. As macrobiotics has long contended, dairy food is a main cause of breast cancer. The Nurses' Health Study II found premenopausal women who ate a lot of high-fat dairy products (like whole milk or butter) had an increased risk of breast cancer.[97] Researchers in California reported breast cancer patients who eat a singe portion of cheese, yogurt, or ice cream daily could be 50% more likely to die. Scientists from the Kaiser Permanente research center in California looked at the records of 1,500 women diagnosed with breast cancer between 1997 and 2000 and concluded that the hormone estrogen found in milk and other dairy products encourages tumor growth.[98]

The BRCA genes are genes that repair chromosomal damage in DNA double-strand breaks. The more milk, cheese, and dairy consumed, the more genetic abnormalities arise, Jack theorized, causing the BRCA repair genes to work harder to repair them. Eventually they become impeded or worn out, mutated, and become ineffective. Scandinavians and the Dutch are well-known consumers of dairy food. In the case of those of Ashkenazi Jewish descent, bagels and cream cheese, cheese blintzes, cheesecake, and cottage cheese, originated in Central and Eastern Europe and were Ashkenazi staples.

From an epigenetic perspective, it appears excessive milk, cheese, and other dairy intake caused hypermethylation or abnormal histone changes at the gene level that were passed along from mother to daughter. Today, BRCA mutations are found in tiny percentages in people of virtually all backgrounds and nationalities, including African-Americans, Native Americans, Pakistanis, and Japanese. By observing the modern food pattern, high in dairy and other cancer-promoting foods such as sugar, women around the world are developing similar epigenetic changes for the worse.[99]

Colon Cancer

Along with lung cancer, colon cancer is the most deadly malignancy for both men and women. In addition to a balanced, plant-based diet, special remedies may be effective to help relieve this condition.

☤ Daikon a Potent Food for Colon Cancer

Daikon, the large white radish used in traditional Far Eastern cooking, has chemopreventive properties. In a study published in the *Journal of Agriculture and Food Chemistry*, researchers reported that an extract of daikon inhibited three lines of human colon cancer cells. Daikon is used regularly in macrobiotic cooking. For many years, educator Michio Kushi has recommended a special Daikon Carrot Drink to help relieve colon cancer and other malignancies. Native to the East, daikon is now grown in North America, Europe, and throughout the world.[100]

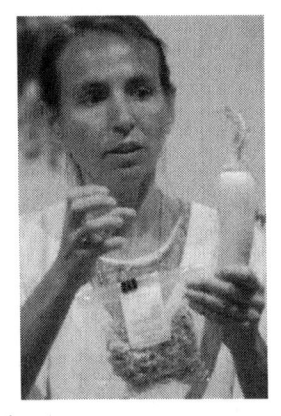

Bettina Zumdick shows the healing properties of daikon radish

Endometrial Cancer

Soy foods are high in isoflavones, naturally occurring compounds that protect from illness. Many medical studies have shown that a diet high in traditionally processed soy (as opposed to soy supplements, analogues, and GMO soy) reduce the risk for female disorders, including endometrial conditions, breast cancer, and reproductive disorders.

☤ Tofu and Legumes May Reduce Endometrial Cancer Risk

Phytochemicals in tofu, legumes, and other soy and legume products reduce the risk of endometrial cancer. University of Hawaii Cancer Center researchers observed 489 non-hysterectomized postmenopausal women with this malignancy over 13.6 years. Reduce endometrial cancer risk was associated with total isoflavone intake, and increasing intake of

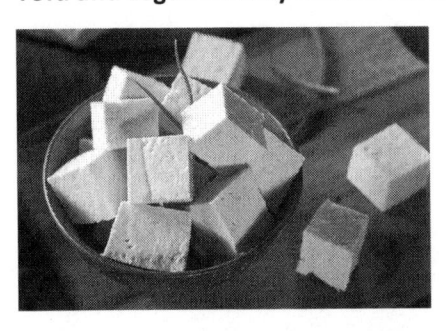

Tofu is a protein-rich soy product that is good for both daily health and for healing

45

tofu or soy did not increase risk.[101] The macrobiotic way has also been helpful for women suffering from endometriosis.

Lung Cancer
Miso and other traditionally made soy foods may help prevent or relieve lung cancer.

☤ Miso Soup and Other Soy Foods Inhibit Lung Cancer
In Japan, soy is consumed in a wide variety of forms, such as miso soup and soy sauce. In a study to investigate the effect of genistein, an isoflavone found in soy, on osteosarcoma cells, Japanese researchers reported in 2012 that miso and other soy foods high in genistein inhibited cell proliferation, especially in the lungs. It decreased invasive and motile potential by inducing cell differentiation. "Genistein may be useful as an anti-metastatic drug for osteosarcoma," the researchers concluded.[102]

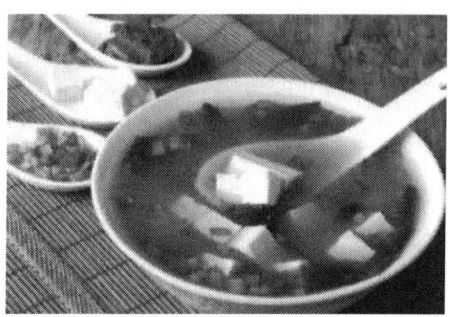

Miso inhibits tumor development

Pancreatic Cancer
Pancreatic cancer has the poorest prognosis of all major types of cancer. As the cases of Jean Kohler, Norman Arnold, and others noted above show, it has lent itself to macrobiotic recoveries. The following medical study was inspired by these successes:

☤ Pancreatic Patients Live Nearly 3 Times Longer
Researchers at Tulane University reported that the 1-year survival rate among patients with pancreatic cancer was significantly higher among those who adopted a macrobiotic diet than among those who did not (17 months versus 6 months). The one-year survival rate was 54.2 percent in the macrobiotic patients versus 10.0 percent in the controls. "This exploratory analysis suggests that a strict macrobiotic diet is more likely to be effective in the long-term management of cancer than are diets that provide a variety of other foods," the scientists concluded in the *American Journal of Clinical Nutrition*.[103]

Prostate Cancer

Prostate cancer is the most prevalent cancer in American men. In addition to several well publicized accounts of personal recoveries, the macrobiotic approach has been studied by several medical researchers:

☤ Prostate Patients Live Nearly Twice as Long

Tulane University researchers found that patients with metastatic prostate cancer who followed a macrobiotic diet lived longer (177 months compared to 91 months) and enjoyed an improved quality of life than controls. The researchers concluded that the macrobiotic approach could be an effective adjunctive treatment to conventional treatment or in primary management of cancers with a nutritional association. "This exploratory analysis suggests that a strict macrobiotic diet is more likely to be effective in the long-term management of cancer than are diets that provide a variety of other foods," the study published in the *American Journal of Nutrition* concluded.[104]

☤ PSA Levels Drop Significantly on a Macrobiotic Diet

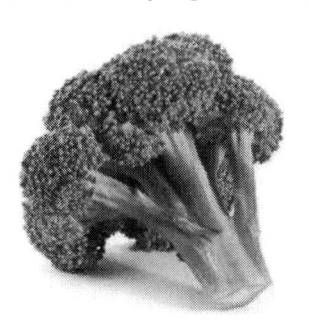

Green vegetables help protect against prostate cancer

At Moores Cancer Center, University of California, San Diego, researchers undertook two intervention studies of patients with recurrent prostate cancer. In a 6-month pilot clinical trial to investigate whether adoption of a modified macrobiotic diet high in whole grains, fresh vegetables, and other plant foods, reinforced by stress management training, could attenuate the rate of further rise of PSA [prostate-specific antigen, a risk factor], 14 patients with recurrent prostate cancer experienced a significant decrease in the rate of PSA rise. Four of 10 evaluable patients experienced an absolute reduction in their PSA levels, nine of ten had a reduction in their rates of PSA rise and improvement of their PSA doubling times. Mean PSA doubling time increased from 11.9 months to 112.3 months. "These results provide preliminary evidence that adoption of a plant-based [macrobiotic] diet, in combination with stress reduction, may attenuate disease progression and have therapeutic potential for clinical management of recurrent prostate cancer," the researchers reported in *Integrative Cancer Therapies* in 2006.[105]

Stomach Cancer
Stomach tumors are linked to eating salted meats, white rice, and other foods in the modern Asian diet where this cancer is widespread.

☤ Miso Protects Against Stomach Cancer and Heart Disease
Japan's National Cancer Center reported that people who eat miso soup daily are 33 percent less likely to contract stomach cancer and have 19 percent less cancer at other sites than those who never eat miso soup. The thirteen-year study, involving about 265,000 men and women over forty, also found that those who never ate miso soup had a 43 percent higher death rate from coronary heart disease than those who consumed miso soup daily. Those who abstained from miso also had 29 percent more fatal strokes, 3.5 times more deaths resulting from high blood pressure, and higher mortality from all other causes.[106]

☤ Shiitake Have Strong Anti-Tumor Effect

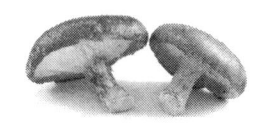

Shiitake help discharge fat and oil deposits in the body and prevent tumors

Japanese scientists at the National Cancer Center Research Institute reported that shiitake mushrooms had a strong anti-tumor effect. In experiments with mice, polysaccharide preparations from various natural sources, including the shiitake mushroom commonly available in Tokyo markets, markedly inhibited the growth of induced sarcomas resulting in "almost complete regression of tumors . . with no sign of toxicity."[107]

General Medical Opinion
As a result of the above studies on the macrobiotic approach to cancer, major medical organizations have generally supported its potential to help prevent and, in some cases, relieve cancer:

☤ American Cancer Society Lists Benefits of Macrobiotics
In a statement on alternative therapies in 1996, the American Cancer Society observed, "Today's most popular anticancer diet is probably macrobiotics." While no diet has yet been shown to be able to reverse existing tumors, the ACS went on: "Like other fat-reducing diets, macrobiotics may help prevent some cancers. It may reduce the risk of developing cancers that appear related to higher fat intake, such as colon cancer and possibly some breast cancers. The macrobiotic diet, like other fat-free diets, can lower blood pressure and perhaps reduce the

chance of heart disease. Taking part in a macrobiotics program may provide some sense of balance with nature and harmony with the total universe and as such promote a sense of calmness and reduced stress."[108]

☤ ACS Says Macrobiotics Assists Conventional Treatment

In advice to cancer survivors, the American Cancer Society further declared in 2003 that the macrobiotic way of eating could be beneficial. "The macrobiotic diet and lifestyle is not primarily aimed at cancer survivors, yet many persons first encounter this diet in the context of cancer. This diet is based on whole grains, vegetables, sea vegetables, beans, fermented soy products, fruit, nuts, seeds, soups, small amounts of fish, and teas. Individualized diets are based on whether a cancer is classified yin or yang. Macrobiotic diets may be used as an adjuvant to conventional treatment to ensure nutritional variety and adequacy."[109]

☤ ACS Recommends a Plant-Based Diet

The American Cancer Society's *Guidelines on Nutrition and Physical Activity for Cancer-Prevention* stated that one-third of malignancies were due to diet and physical activity habits. Among its key recommendations were "Consume a healthy diet, with an emphasis on plant foods," "Choose whole grains instead of refined grain products," "Limit consumption of processed meat and red meat."[110]

☤ Macrobiotic Diet Improves Drug Metabolism

In a review of complementary and alternative therapies for cancer in *American Family Physician*, a researcher reported that a macrobiotic diet may positively alter drug metabolism and that in well-nourished patients who do not have breast or endometrial cancer, "a macrobiotic diet can be accepted by the physician as an adjunct of conventional treatment."[111]

As these studies indicate, macrobiotics opened the way for research on the dietary approach to cancer. Michio Kushi met with Dr. Mark Hegsted, a nutritionalist from Harvard, and others who influenced *Dietary Goals for the U.S.*, the historic 1977 Senate report linking the modern way of eating with heart disease, cancer, and other leading causes of death and led to the first national and international dietary guidelines for cancer. In the years that followed, macrobiotics became the most popular dietary treatment for those with this disease. Every year, these recommendations move closer to the macrobiotic approach. For example, the American Cancer Society dietary guidelines for cancer emphasizing a plant-based approach noted above were composed in 2012 by a committee chaired by Lawrence H. Kushi, ScD, an epidemiologist and breast cancer researcher, son of Michio and Aveline Kushi, and lifelong practitioner of macrobiotics.[112]

AIDS

In 1983 a group of young men in New York City with AIDS began macrobiotics under the guidance of Michio Kushi. They hoped to change their blood quality, recover their natural immunity, and survive at that time a nearly always fatal illness. In May, 1984, a research team led by Martha C. Cottrell, M.D., Director of Student Health at the Fashion Institute of Technology in New York, Elinor N. Levy, Ph.D. and John C. Beldekas, Ph.D. of the Department of Immunology and Microbiology at Boston University's School of Medicine, began to monitor the blood samples and immune functions of ten men with Kaposi's sarcoma (a usual symptom of AIDS). They issued a series of reports on their findings. The macrobiotic approach to AIDS was outlined in *AIDS, Macrobiotics, and Natural Immunity* by Michio Kushi and Martha Cottrell, M.D., *AIDS & Diet* by Kushi and Alex Jack, and *The Way of Hope: Michio Kushi's Anti-AIDS Program* by Tom Monte.

☤ Men with AIDS Stabilize on Macrobiotics

The NYC research team reported in *Lancet*, the British medical journal, that the men with AIDS were stabilizing on the macrobiotic diet. "Survival in these men who have received little or no medical treatment appears to compare very favorably with that of KS [Kaposi's sarcoma] patients in general. We suggest that physicians and scientists can feel comfortable in allowing patients, particularly those with minimal disease, to go untreated as part of a larger [dietary] study or because non-treatment is the patient's choice."[113]

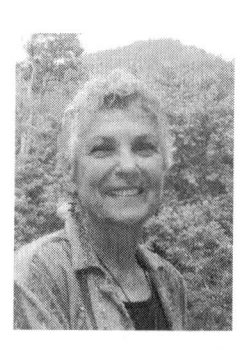

Martha C. Cottrell, M.D. led the macrobiotic AIDS project in New York

☤ Modern Agriculture Led to Evolution of HIV

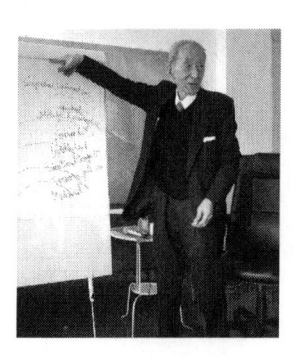

Michio Kushi led a seminar on diet and AIDS in the Republic of the Congo

In an analysis of diet and immune-deficiency disorders, educator Michio Kushi, who led an AIDS and diet seminar for 250 medical doctors in Africa sponsored by the World Health Organization (WHO), attributed the emergence of HIV and other new viruses to modern agricultural practices and patterns of food consumption that have disrupted traditional societies and ecosystems that have existed in harmony for thousands of years. HIV acquired its virulence and elusiveness as a result of modern environmental and medical interventions, including monocropping, pesticide and chemical fertilizer use, and abuse of antibiotics and other drugs. As it made its way through depleted soil, a chemically weakened food chain, and immuno-suppressed blood systems, HIV gradually evolved into a stronger, more lethal virus. Kushi also explored the role that a modern diet based on extremely expansive foods such as sugar, sweets, fatty foods, oily and greasy foods, and fruits and juices, as well as use of too much alcohol, drugs, and medications, may have played in loss of natural immunity to disease.[114]

☤ Umeboshi Plums Protect Against H1N1 Virus.

Umeboshi, an aged, salted, pickled plum and staple in macrobiotic cooking, contain a substance that can suppress the growth of the H1N1 virus, researchers at the Wakayama Medical University in Japan reported. They said the substance is a type of polyphenol whose existence has not been previously confirmed. When applied to the affected cells, the growth of the virus was suppressed by roughly 90 percent after about seven hours. "We can expect to suppress the virus growth by having about five pieces of umeboshi a day," Hirotoshi Utsunomiya, associate professor of pathology and team leader, said. Ume-Sho-Bancha and Ume-Sho-Kuzu medicinal drinks are two of the main macrobiotic home remedies for preventing or relieving swine flu and other infectious conditions.[115]

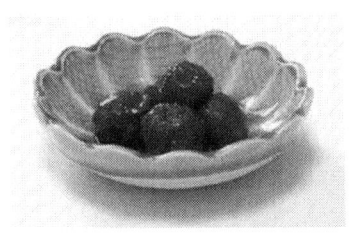

Umeboshi plums protect against infection and strengthen the blood

Arthritis

Arthritis, a painful bone and joint disease, affects millions of people. Major forms include osteoarthritis, the painful hardening of bones and joints in the hands or spine, which affects primarily older people, especially men. Rheumatoid arthritis, involving the inflammation and swelling of the joints, especially in the hands and feet, appears primarily in women aged 25 to 50. A balanced diet has benefited many people with arthritis. In macrobiotic counseling experience, excessive animal food and salt contributes to osteoarthritis, while potatoes, tomatoes, and other nightshade plants may lead to rheumatoid arthritis.

☤ Vegan Diet Improves Symptoms of Rheumatoid Arthritis

In a random case-control study of 66 patients with active rheumatoid arthritis, scientists reported that 40% of the vegan diet group experienced improvement compared to 4% of the group eating a nonvegan diet. "The immunoglobulin G (IgG) antibody levels against gliadin and beta-lactoglobulin decreased in the responder subgroup in the vegan diet-treated patients, but not in the other analysed groups." The researchers concluded that the vegan diet (which avoids all animal products and emphasizes whole grains, vegetables, and other plant quality foods) may be of benefit to certain RA patients.[116]

☤ Traditional Societies Free of Arthritis

"Arthritis is not a genetic disease, nor is it an inevitable part of growing older—there are causes for these joint afflictions, and they lie in our environment—our closest contact with our environment is our food," explains Dr. John McDougall, an American holistic medical doctor. He cites research showing that rheumatoid arthritis did not exist before 1800 and that many types of arthritis were rare to nonexistent in rural regions of Africa and Asia. "As recently as 1957, no case of rheumatoid arthritis could be found in Africa. That was a time when people in Africa followed diets based on grains and vegetables." However, with the influx of meat, dairy products, and highly processed foods, arthritis began to appear in traditional societies. "An unhealthy diet containing dairy and other animal products causes inflammation of the intestinal surfaces and thereby increases the passage of dietary and/or bacterial antigens," Dr. McDougall observed.[117]

☤ Nightshades Linked to Arthritis

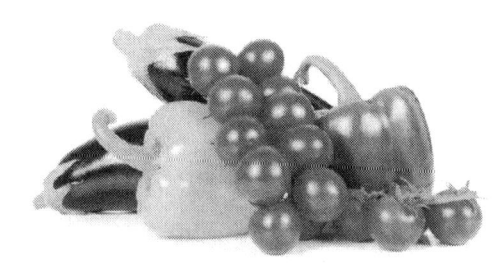

Tomatoes, potatoes, eggplant, peppers, and other members of the nightshade family are a principal cause of arthritis. In a survey of over 1400 persons over a 20-year period, researchers at Rutgers University, the University of Florida, and the Arthritis Nightshades Research Foundation reported that these plants, along with tobacco (another member of the nightshade family) are an important causative factor in arthritis in sensitive people. "Osteoarthritis appears to be a result of long-term consumption and/or use of the Solanaceae which contain naturally the active metabolite, vitamin D3, which in excess causes crippling and early disability (as seen in livestock)." Removing nightshades from the diet has "resulted in positive to marked improvement in arthritis and general health," the researchers concluded in the *Journal of Neurological and Orthopedic Medical Surgery*.[118]

Autism

Autism, in which the child does not develop close personal relationships and lives in a world of their own, usually appears between one and three, and symptoms persist throughout life. Medically, autism is considered irreversible.

⚕ Sonic Rebirth

Simulating the sound of the mother's voice in utero, Alfred Tomatis, M.D., the French expert on the effects of sound and music on human development, has helped relieve many cases of autism by recreating the sound of the mother's voice in embryo and playing it back to the autistic child to reestablish the sonic contact that was disrupted in the womb. "The vocal nourishment that the mother provides is just as important as her milk," he explains. For adopted children or children whose mother is dead or incapacitated, he uses the filtered music of Mozart, which has a similar effect. Dr. Tomatis recommends a natural diet high in whole grains, fresh vegetables, and less dairy food, especially yogurt, for optimal hearing and development.[119]

☙ Boy Recovers from Autism with Macrobiotics and Music

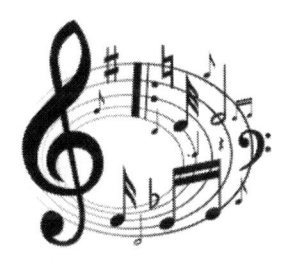

Judy and Dick Harvey adopted James, an orphan from Vietnam who was later diagnosed as autistic, in the early 1970s. The boy loved to eat french fries, cheese, candy, and salty foods, but discontinued these, along with dairy, red meat, eggs, poultry, and refined sugar following a consultation with educator Michio Kushi. Through macrobiotics and participation in classical music, he overcame his disabilities, went on to study at the University of Nebraska where he majored in math and physics, and is now living a normal life.[120]

☙ Autistic Girl Changes Diet and Tests Normal within a Year

After only two weeks on a macrobiotic diet, parents of an autistic little girl noticed positive changes. (The family chose to remain anonymous.) Almost daily she emerged with new skills. A year later, she was a completely different child. "Her therapists and teachers were all amazed by how much she has changed and progressed," the parents related. "When retested for speech, her scores were well above the average for her age. The only trace of autism was her pragmatic speech, and difficulty coming up with new ideas to maintain a dialog with peers. But that too was continually and rapidly improving. Incredibly, within a year she was at the level of a typically-developing child in the following ways: 1) eye contact, 2) joint attention, 3) the desire and initiative for social interaction and play with peers, 4) the ability to show and recognize a wide variety of emotions and appropriately respond to them, 5) pretend play skills."[121]

☤ Gluten- and Dairy-Free Diets Reduce Autistic Behavior

In a review of nutritional approaches to autism, researchers at the Center for Reading Research at Stravanger University College in Norway reported that gluten and/or casein (dairy) free diets help reduce autistic behavior, increase social and communicative skills, and lead to the reappearance of autistic traits if the children go off the diet. In a randomized double-blind study of 20 autistic children, researchers in Norway found that children given a diet low in gluten, gliadin, and casein (dairy protein) developed significantly better than controls.[122]

Celiac Disease

Celiac disease (DC) is a genetic disorder of the small intestine. Exposure to wheat, barley, rye, and other gluten products causes an inflammatory response that atrophies the villi and interferes with absorption. CD was first described in the 1880s and linked to wheat only in the 1940s. While the disorder is hard to reverse, a macrobiotic way of eating, centered on rice, millet, and other non-glutenous grains, usually improves digestion. *See Gluten Intolerance below.*

☙ Refining of Wheat May Underlie Celiac

For thousands of years, wheat, barley, and other glutinous foods were consumed as staple foods without any reported intolerances or digestive problems. The emergence of Celiac in the late 19th century accompanied the refining of grains that made cheap white bread widely available. According to macrobiotic researcher Alex Jack, consumption of excessive refined flour and other adulterated gluten products may have led to a gene mutation

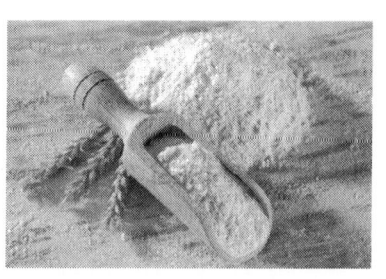

The refining of white flour coincided with the rise of Celiac Disease and gluten intolerance

that was inheritable among susceptible family members. A similar process appears to have led to the mutation of the BRCA gene linked to breast cancer following increased dairy consumption in Europe. In the case of Celiac, the villi of the small intestine appear to have lost the ability to function properly after excessive exposure to refined flour, especially that made with commercial baker's yeast and other additives.[123]

Children's Health

Nutritionists and physicians initially raised questions about the adequacy of the macrobiotic regimen for children, especially since they were not getting dairy products. But over the years, scientific and medical studies generally found that macrobiotic youngsters were adequately nourished and in many cases exceeded the nutritional levels of ordinary children eating the modern way.

☤ Macrobiotic Day-Care Center a Model for British Children

A British nutritionist found that a macrobiotic day-care center in London not only "supported normal growth" in nursery school children but also could be used as a model to implement national dietary guidelines. Comparing the nutritional adequacy of macrobiotic meals provided preschool children by the Community Health Foundation with ordinary meals at a nursery in Notting Hill, the investigator found that the macrobiotic food met current U.K.-R.D.I. dietary, energy, and nutrient standards and that the children's anthropometric measurements including weight, height, and skinfold thicknesses were normal. In contrast, the ordinary nursery school diet was high in dairy food, lard, and other saturated fats that have been associated with the development of atherosclerosis beginning in childhood. "This illustrates the power and potential of nursery meals to contribute to the adoption of a nutritionally sound and beneficial national diet."[124]

☤ Macrobiotic Children Develop Normally

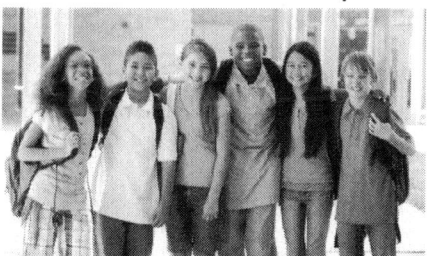

Macrobiotic children test healthy and have higher IQs than other kids

In a study of vegetarian preschool children, researchers at New England Medical Center Hospital in Boston found that the growth of macrobiotic youngsters did not significantly differ from those of non-macrobiotics before age two. After age two, macrobiotic children tended to put on weight more quickly than the children brought up on yoga diets, Seventh-Day Adventist diets, or other vegetarian regimes. Nearly all the children had been breast-fed, and it was found that macrobiotic children who had been weaned did not differ in caloric intake from non-macrobiotics, according to the study published in *Pediatrics*.[125]

⚕ Macrobiotic Children Have Higher IQs

In a study of mental development, macrobiotic and vegetarian children were brighter and more intelligent than ordinary youngsters their age. The mean I.Q. was 116 for the group as a whole, or 16 percent above average. The children's mean mental age was found to exceed their mean chronologic age by approximately a year. The macrobiotic children's I.Q.'s and mental ages were slightly higher than the other vegetarians. "In the judgments of both the pediatrician and psychologic technician, the children as a group were bright," the researchers concluded in the *Journal of the Amercian Dietetic Association*. They speculated, however, that the brightness may be due to better education on the part of the macrobiotic and vegetarian parents, not to diet.[126]

Crohn's Disease

Crohn's Disease is an inflammatory bowel disease for which there is no medical cure. However, it lends itself to improvement or recovery with a macrobiotic diet.

↷ Free of Crohn's for 35 Years

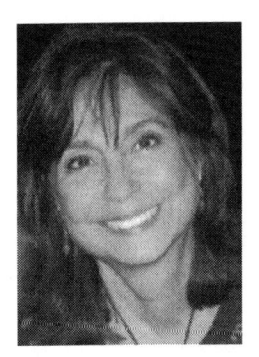

After suffering for seven years from Crohn's, Virginia Harper recovered with the help of macrobiotics. Over the last 35 years, she has enjoyed optimal health and gone on to become a leading macrobiotic teacher and counselor. At You Can Heal You, her healing center in Nashville, Virginia has helped many others with digestive disorders and teaches worldwide. She is the author of *Controlling Crohn's the Natural Way*.[127]

After recovering, Virginia Harper guided many others to greater health

Diabetes

Nearly 30 million Americans—1 in 8—are diagnosed with diabetes, the fastest growing chronic disease in the country, and nearly 300 million people around the globe have the condition. According to the World Health Organization (WHO), the number of cases will double by 2030. Special programs on a dietary approach to diabetes were offered at Kushi Institute and other macrobiotic centers. In Italy, the International Un Punto Macrobiotico Foundation sponsored diabetes intervention studies in Thailand, Cuba, and other countries. Planetary Health, Inc. proposed a macrobiotic study for the Middle East, where diabetes is skyrocketing, and published a primer *Diabetes: The Macrobiotic Approach*.

▼ Thai Patients Get Off Insulin on Macrobiotic Diet

A study by the Ministry of Public Health in Thailand found that a macrobiotic way of eating (known as the Ma-Pi 2 Diet) designed by Italian educator Mario Pianesi offers an effective, alternate approach to the care of diabetes patients and that it may help patients on insulin maintain their blood sugar levels without an insulin injection. In a dietary intervention study at the Wanakaset Research Facility of Kasetart University in Trad Province, researchers found a statistically significant reduction in blood sugar levels, weight, blood pressure, and heartbeat ratios among 44 patients put on a macrobiotic way of eating. "Subjects were in significantly better health, more vibrant, more peaceful, and more energetic," the study reported in 2006. The four patients on insulin were able to maintain their blood sugar levels within the range of 110-171 mg without any insulin injections and all subjects were free of any adverse effects.[128]

▼ Cuban Patients Get Off Insulin

In a 6-month macrobiotic dietary intervention study of the Ma-Pi 2 Diet carried out in 16 adults with Type 2 diabetes at the Diabetic Care Center in Colon, Cuban physicians reported in 2009 that anthropometric variables significantly improved, including lean body mass and glucide and lipid metabolism. "All participants were able to eliminate insulin treatment, and 25 percent continued treatment with glibenclamide only," the researchers reported. "According to lipid levels and ratios, cardiovascular risk was also considerably reduced." The investigators noted. "Hemoglobin, total protein, albumin, and creatinin levels indicated that nutritional safety was maintained. There were no adverse events."[129]

▼ Brown Rice Consumption Reduces Diabetes Risk

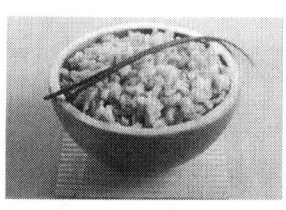

Researchers from the Harvard School of Public Health (HSPH) have found that eating five or more servings of white rice per week was associated with an increased risk of type 2 diabetes. In contrast, eating two or more servings of brown rice per week was associated with a lower risk of the disease. The researchers estimated that replacing 50 grams of white rice (just one third of a typical daily serving) with the same amount of brown rice would lower risk of type 2 diabetes by 16%. The same replacement with other whole grains, such as whole wheat and barley, was associated with a 36% reduced risk.[130]

Harvard researchers say whole grains can reduce diabetes by up to 36%

⚕ American Patients Get Off or Reduce Insulin

In a review of the macrobiotic approach to diabetes, Robert H. Lerman, M.D., Ph.D. cited a recent case series in 13 patients with type 2 diabetes provided with nutrition education and provided with meals at the Kushi Institute. Under the supervision of Martha Cottrell, M.D., most experienced reduction in or elimination of diabetes medication, weight loss, reduced blood pressure, and improvement in energy after starting the new way of eating in the course of the program.[131]

Ebola

Following the outbreak of Ebola in 2014, the macrobiotic community prepared dietary guidelines for the epidemic then raging in West Africa.

Modern Agriculture Linked to New Viral Diseases

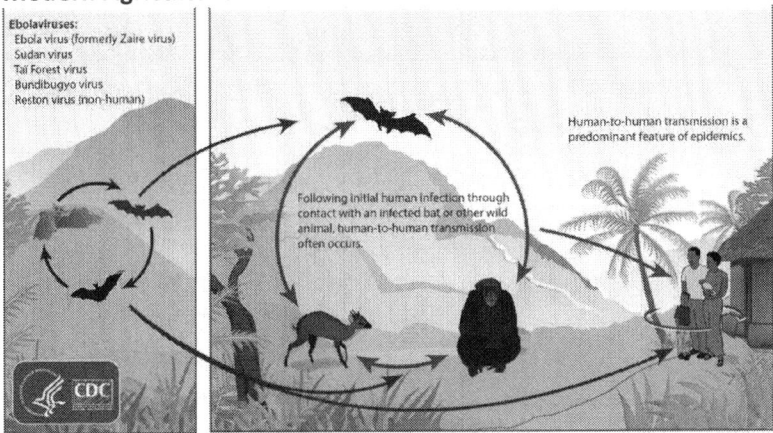

In consultation with Michio Kushi, Planetary Health researchers Alex Jack, Edward Esko, and Sachi Kato hypothesized that Ebola broke out in Central Africa following the introduction of monoculture and commodity crops, especially cassava and bananas, which displaced grains, beans, and other organic and natural crops. The changes upset the delicate checks and balances in the soil biota and in local ecosystems, giving rise to virulent new strains of microorganisms. After coming into contact with chimpanzees or other primates infected with Ebola virus, SIV (Simian Immune-deficiency Virus, the precursor to HIV), and other pathogens or eating contaminated bushmeat, people in this region acquired natural immune deficiency, and Marburg (1967), Ebola (1976), AIDS (1981), and other lethal diseases took hold and spread. In the case of Ebola, the virus originated with contaminated fruit that was eaten by bats and passed to primates and humans. The potency of the virus increased with each mammal and compounded its virulence. The guidelines, including home remedies to treat symptoms, appeared on www.ebolaanddiet.com and helped airlines personnel, travelers, and others in the region deal with the emergency.[132]

Environmental Illness

Macrobiotics has been helpful in dealing with environmental illness and chemical sensitivity.

⚕ Physician Heals E.I. with Macrobiotic Diet

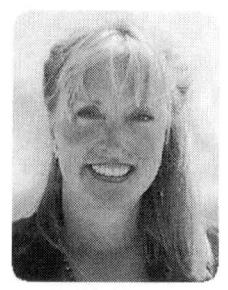

Sherry Rogers, M.D. used diet to recover from severe chemical sensitivities

In 1974 Sherry A. Rogers, M.D., a 31-year-old physician, suffered from Environmental Illness. She had ugly red eczema over the lower half of her face, periodic asthma, recurrent sinus problems, wicked migraines, chronic back pain from an old riding injury, and unwarranted exhaustion and depression. By the early 1980s she was having strong adverse reactions to chemicals such as workmen gluing down a new Formica countertop. She had treated her sensitivities with injections, multiple vitamins and ionizers, cotton blankets and pillows, bottled water, oxygen tanks, aluminum foil. In 1987, after following a macrobiotic diet for six months, the excruciating shoulder pain disappeared, and over the next few months other chronic symptoms vanished.[133]

⚕ Diet Helps Patients Suffering from Chemical Sensitivity

In a study of 160 patients suffering from chemical sensitivity, those who followed a macrobiotic diet for at least one year reported an average decrease in chemical sensitivity of 76 percent, according to an article in the *Journal of Applied Nutrition*.[134]

Geriatrics

The term "macrobiotics" means long life, and a balanced, whole foods diet has traditionally been associated with healthy aging and prolonging life. In one study in at a Boston hospital, researchers found that geriatric patients experienced significant improvement on a macrobiotic diet.

⚕ Macrobiotics Assists Psychiatric and Geriatric Patients

Dr. Jonathan Lieff, Chief of Psychiatry and Geriatric Services at the Shattuck Hospital in Boston and doctors at Tufts University School of Nutrition, designed an experiment in 1982 to test the effect of macrobiotic food on long-term psychiatric and geriatric patients. Some of these people had been confined in the hospital for 30 years or more. In a double-blind study in which neither the ordinary hospital staff or patients knew they were participating, macrobiotic meals avoiding meat, sugar, processed foods, and synthetic food additives and including whole grains, legumes, fresh vegetables and fruits designed to look and taste like regular foods were introduced to a ward of 16 patients over an eight-week period and 18 controls. Altogether 187 food items on the macrobiotic menu were prepared, as well as chicken, coffee, and butter which were difficult to simulate. During the test, the researchers noted medically significant reductions in psychosis and agitation among the patients. The scientists found significant improvement in experimental group cooperativeness when compared to the control group, as well as less irritability and improvement upon manifest psychosis. "These data show that the described change in total diet does have a significantly favorable effect on the health and behavior of geropsychiatric patients," the observers concluded.[135]

Gluten Intolerance

Celiac affects only a tiny fraction of the population, while gluten intolerance affects millions of people. It arose following the introduction of new hybrid varieties of dwarf wheat during the Green Revolution in the 1950s and 1960s. The wheat led to higher yields but required synthetic fertilizers and pesticides and much more water. When switching to organic whole wheat or barley from heirloom seeds, many people with gluten sensitivities are able to digest gluten without difficulty.[136] Macrobiotics has been helpful for many people with gluten sensitivities.

Ex-Gluten Sufferer Changes Diet and Enthuses 'I Love Gluten'

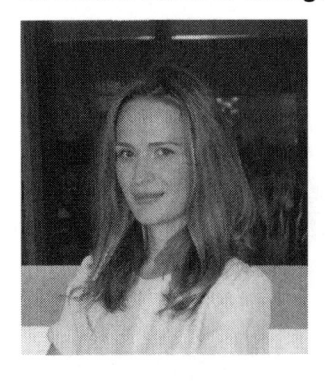

Katya Thomas recovered from crippling gluten intolerance and is now a natural foods cook and healer

Born in Russia, Katya Thomas moved to the Netherlands with her family while she was a teenager. By her early twenties, she had developed severe gluten allergies. Just the taste of a morsel of food containing wheat, barley, or oats would precipitate violent symptoms. Doctors told her that she would have to avoid glutinous products the rest of her life. But on a gluten-free diet, Katya soon discovered that most of the products targeted for people like her contained sugar, chemicals, and other ingredients that only made her condition worse. Determined to heal herself naturally, Katya tried many vegetarian and vegan approaches. Ultimately, a balanced macrobiotic diet not only regularized her digestion, but also enabled her to enjoy wheat and other glutenous foods again. Today she is a natural foods cook, consultant, and healer, and her story "I Love Gluten" and classes have helped others recover from gluten sensitivities.[137]

Hospital Food

The modern hospital diet dates to Fanny Farmer, the popular cookbook author who was the first woman to lecture at Harvard Medical School in the early 20th century. Her medicinal recipes were as bland and tasteless as her ordinary recipes were rich and artery-clogging. Macrobiotics has been introduced into several hospitals and influenced many others to begin to serve whole grains, fresh foods, and other healing foods.

☤ Boston Hospital Serves Macrobiotic Food

In 1980, a macrobiotic lunch program was started at the Lemuel Shattuck Hospital in Boston for doctors, nurses, and staff. Overall response was favorable and improved noticeably after the macrobiotic food line was integrated with the regular cafeteria line. By the second year, half of the food served each day in the cafeteria was prepared macrobiotically. Regular attendance in-Creased from about 60 to 120 to 200 persons each day. At lunch, from 70 to 90 percent of all meals served included at least one item from the macrobiotic menu. Dr. William Castelli, director of the Framingham Heart Study, contrasted the healthfulness of the macrobiotic food program at the Shattuck Hospital with ordinary hospital food.[138]

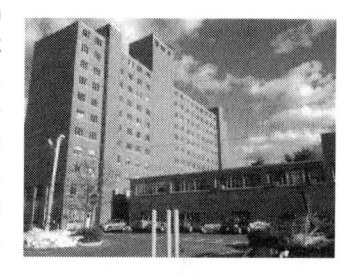

Shattuck Hospital instituted a macrobiotic lunch program

☤ Irish Hospital Offers Macrobiotic Meals

Macrobiotic food was introduced at the National Children's Hospital in Dublin, Ireland. Cecilia Armelin, pediatric dietitian, drew up a sample meal plan including for breakfast: whole oat porridge; for lunch: miso soup with dulse and parsley, brown rice with haricot or azuki beans, Brussels sprouts, dried apricots and raisins; and for dinner: lentil/barley soup seasoned with miso and parsley and whole grain millet with pears and chopped walnuts. She especially recommended these foods for children with multiple allergies or food intolerance.[139]

Medical Education

Until recently, medical schools offered little if any instruction in nutrition. As alternative medicine went mainstream, they began to encourage their students to become familiar with acupuncture, macrobiotics, yoga, and other popular complementary approaches.

⚕ AMA Encourages Students to Sample Macrobiotic Meal

By 1998, the American Medical Association reported that two-thirds of medical schools in the United States were offering courses in alternative and complementary medicine. Among the key recommendations offered by the physicians was that the new medical school curricula include an experiential component. Macrobiotics was singled out in *JAMA* (*Journal of the American Medical Association*) as one of the principal modalities which young medical school students should be familiar with: "Experiencing acupuncture or therapeutic massage or tasting a macrobiotic meal adds a dimension to the learning experience that a lecture or simple demonstration cannot. The deeper understanding that results should provide a better basis for responsibly advising patients."[140]

By 2015, nearly 90% offered courses in alternative medicine, according to the Association of American Medical Colleges.[141]

Mental and Emotional Health

From the macrobiotic view, there is no rigid distinction between mind and body and between spirit and matter. Food governs mental, emotional, and spiritual health as well as physical health and vitality. Individuals and families have overcome a variety of mental and emotional conditions ranging from anxiety and depression to schizophrenia and other severe mental illnesses.

☋ Man Recovers from Schizophrenia with Macrobiotics

With the help of his mother, Charlotte Mahoney-Briscoe, David Briscoe healed himself of schizophrenia by adhering to a balanced macrobiotic diet. David, diagnosed with mental and emotional illness in the 1960s, unsuccessfully tried many hospitals, medications, and confinement before changing his diet. In high school, he become physically ill, with acute kidney problems, frequent sore throats, digestive problems, fevers, and a duodenal ulcer. For his depression, he went to psychiatrists for six years and became addicted to Thorazine. After changing his way of eating to brown rice, soy sauce, and other foods, he made a

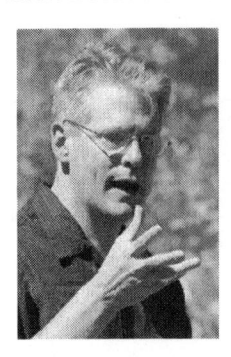

David Briscoe became a leading teacher

complete recovery. David is currently married, the father of four children, and director of Macrobiotics America, an online school.[142]

☤ Diet Effective in Treating Mental Illness

Dr. Stephen Harnish, a New Hampshire psychiatrist, reported that macrobiotics had benefited many of his patients who were chronically and severely mentally ill. Citing several case histories, he described a young woman with a history of severe depression who had been in a state hospital for two years and treated with anti-depressants and antipsychotic medications. Tests by Dr. Harnish's department found that the woman was hypoglycemic and administration of a macrobiotic diet high in complex carbohydrates and one that avoided animal food and sugar resulted in steady improvement, reduced medication, and return to normal functioning. "She now has motivation to do new things and has made plans to return to school." He noted that hundreds of other psychiatric patients could benefit from this approach.[143]

Microwave Cooking

A clean, natural flame is ideal for cooking. Wood, gas, kerosene, charcoal, solar, or other renewable energy source is best. Macrobiotics discourages electrical and microwave cooking that give a chaotic vibration and weaken the food.

☤ Microwaved Food Alters Blood Chemistry

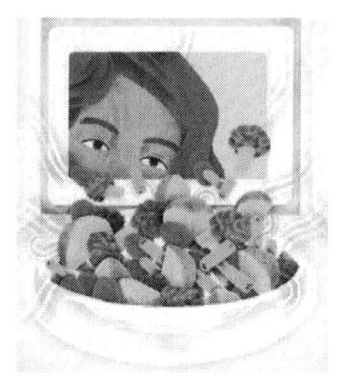

In a study of people eating a macrobiotic diet, researchers at the Swiss Institute of Technology and the University Institute for Biochemistry and the Environmental-Biological Research and Consultation reported that microwaved food produced a decrease in hemoglobin; an increase in hematocrit, and leukocytes; higher cholesterol, and a decrease in lymphocytes. In addition to altering blood chemistry, the researchers found that microwaved food appeared to increase the activity of certain bacteria in the food, and altered cells resembled the pathogenic stages that occur in the early development of some cancers. The scientists also reported biological changes in the microwaved food itself, including increased acidity, damaged protein molecules, enlarged fat cells, and decreased folic acid, a nutrient in the vitamin B group associated with protecting against spina bifida, a birth defect.[144]

Migraine and PMS
Over the years, the East West Foundation, Kushi Institute, and other macrobiotic organizations published case histories of of people who recovered from scores of common conditions ranging from flu and infectious diseases to female disorders, from digestive and circulatory conditions to severe nervous disorders.

⚕ Severe Headaches and Female Complaints Eliminated
A former medical consultant for the Department of National Health and Welfare in Canada successfully treated her own migraine headaches with a macrobiotic diet. Dr. Helen V. Farrell reported that she suffered from classical migraines since she was eleven, experiencing scintillating scotomas, dysplasia, transient parasthesias, and vomiting. As she grew older, the headaches were less frequent, and when she discontinued dairy food and exercised regularly they began to disappear altogether. Dr. Farrell, who specializes in treating female complaints, has successfully introduced many of her patients to a macrobiotic diet. She reports that it is particularly effective in treating premenstrual syndrome.[145]

Nuclear Radiation
From the atomic bombings of Hiroshima and Nagasaki to nuclear accidents in the Soviet Union, macrobiotic quality foods proved instrumental in preventing and relieving atomic sickness, including leukemia, thyroid cancer, and other consequences of excessive exposure to radioactivity. Medical studies in Japan and Canada confirmed the ability of miso and sea vegetables to discharge Cesium-37, Strontium-90, and other radioactive particles from the body. In 1990, the Kushi Institute organized an airlift of thousands of pounds of miso, seaweed, and other major staples to give to Soviet medical doctors in Chelyabinsk and Chernobyl.

⚕ Macrobiotic Diet Saves All Patients in Nagasaki
In August, 1945, at the time of the atomic bombing of Japan, Tatsuichiro Akizuki, M.D., was director of the Department of Internal Medicine at St. Francis's Hospital in Nagasaki. Most patients in the hospital, located one mile from the center of the blast, survived the initial effects of the bomb, but soon after came down with symptoms of radiation sickness from the fallout that had been released. Dr. Akizuki fed his staff and patients a strict macrobiotic diet of brown rice, miso soup, wakame and other sea vegeta-

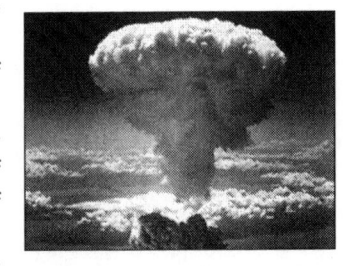

All patients at St. Francis Hospital in Naasaki survived atomic sickness on a macrobiotic diet

bles, Hokkaido pumpkin, and sea salt and prohibited the consumption of sugar and sweets. As a result, he saved everyone in his hospital, while many other survivors in the city perished from radiation sickness. "I gave the cooks and staff strict orders that they should make unpolished whole-grain rice balls, adding some salt to them, prepare strong miso soup for each meal, and never use sugar. When they didn't follow my orders, I scolded them without mercy, 'Never take sugar. Sugar will destroy your blood!'. . ."This dietary method made it possible for me to remain alive and go on working vigorously as a doctor. . . . It was thanks to this food that all of us could work for people day after day, overcoming fatigue or symptoms of atomic disease and survive the disaster free from severe symptoms of radioactivity."[146]

Miso Soup Key Food in Protecting Against Nuclear Fallout

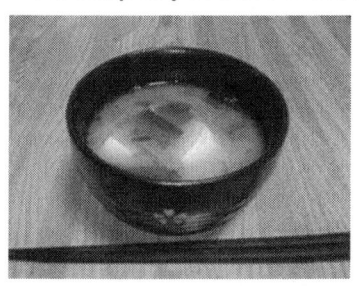

Atomic bomb survivors credited miso with helping to prevent radiation sickness

In interviews sixty years after the atomic bombing of Japan, seven former patients at St. Francis Hospital, fourteen other atomic survivors in Nagasaki, and eight survivors in Hiroshima described how miso soup and other macrobiotic quality foods helped them prevent or relieve radiation sickness. Analyzing her findings, Hiroko Furo, an associate professor at Illinois Wesleyan University, concluded that "miso was very helpful for the survivors' healing and that macrobiotic food contributed to the easing atomic bomb syndrome." Dr. Furo suggested that the macrobiotic diet would be useful for those who are undergoing radiation therapy and may eventually be incorporated into the medical treatment of cancer.[147]

Kelp Protects Against Nuclear Fallout and Radiation

During the Cold War, scientists at the Gastro-Intestinal Research Laboratory at McGill University in Montreal, Canada, reported that a substance derived from the sea vegetable kelp could reduce by 50 to 80 percent the amount of radioactive strontium absorbed through the intestine. Stanley Skoryna, M.D. said in the *Canadian Medical Journal* in 1964 that in animal experiments sodium alginate obtained from brown algae permitted calcium to be normally absorbed through the intestinal wall while binding most of the strontium. The sodium alginate and strontium were subsequently excreted from the body. The experiments were designed to devise a method to counteract the effects of fallout and radiation.[148]

☤ Miso Eliminates Deadly Iodine-131 from the Body

Following up the macrobiotic survivals in Hiroshima and Nagasaki from radition sickness at the end of World War II, Japanese reseachers reported that miso is effective in helping to remove radioactive elements from the body and controlling inflammation of organs caused by radioactivity. In laboratory studies, researchers at Hiroshima University Medical Center found that there was only half the amount of radioactive iodine 131 in the blood of the group of rats fed with miso in contrast to the control group three and six hours after the injections. Lower amounts of radioactive particles were also measured in the kidneys, liver, and spleen. Although there was no difference in the amount of radioactive cesium in the blood, a high amount of cesium was eliminated from the muscles of the group eating miso.[149]

☤ Macrobiotic Diet Helps Victims of Soviet Nuclear Accidents

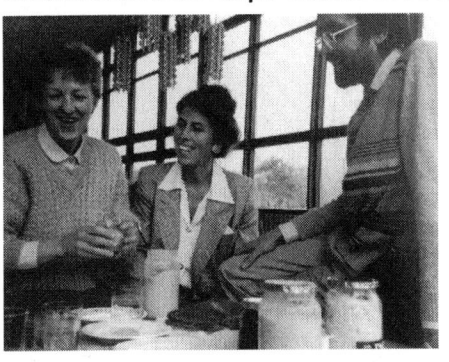

Lidia Yamchuk and Hanif Shaimardanov, medical doctors in Cheljabinsk, organized Longevity, the first macrobiotic association in the Soviet Union in 1985. At their hospital, they used dietary methods and acupuncture to treat many patients, especially those suffering from leukemia, lymphoma, and other disorders associated with exposure to nuclear radiation. Since the early 1950s, wastes from Soviet weapons production were dumped into Karachay Lake in Cheljabinsk, an industrial city about 900 miles east of Moscow that was the center for Soviet nuclear weapons production during the Cold War. In Leningrad, Yuri Stavitsky, a young pathologist and medical instructor, volunteered as a radiologist in Chernobyl after the nuclear accident on April 26, 1986. Since then, like many disaster workers, he suffered symptoms associated with radiation disease, including tumors of the thyroid. "Since beginning macrobiotics," he reported, "my condition has greatly improved."[150]

Soviet physicians Lidia Yamchuk (left) and Hanif Shaimardanov (right) used macrobiotics to help heal victims of nuclear accidents. Macrobiotic teacher Cary Wolf, part of a delegation from the Kushi Institute in America that donated thousands of pounds of miso, sea vegetables, and other natural foods, is in the center

Obesity

Two out of three American adults and one out of three children are overweight or obese. These are major risk factors for diabetes, heart disease, selected cancers, and other disorders. Almost everyone who starts macrobiotics loses weight as green protein and polyunsaturated fats and oils replace animal-quality protein and saturated fat. The Kushi Institute instituted a popular Weight-Loss Seminar and macrobiotic counselors and personal chefs were consulted frequently for this condition.

☤ Kanten Key Food in Weight Loss Diet

Kanten, the traditional Japanese gelatin, made from agar-agar seaweed and an important part of the macrobiotic way of eating, is a key food to reduce obesity and chronic disease. In a study of 76 overweight patients given a balanced weight-loss diet, Japanese scientists report that those given a small serving of kanten before their dinner lost 4.4 percent of their body weight over 12 weeks compared to 2.2 percent by controls.[151]

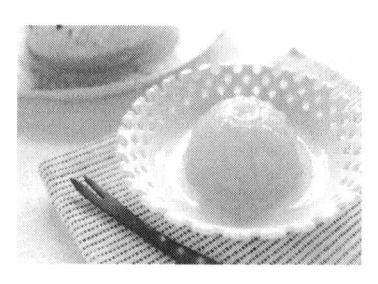

Kanten, a plant-based gelatin, assists in weight loss

Osteoporosis

Osteoporosis, the thinning of the bones and susceptibility to fracture, commonly occurs in middle aged and elderly people as a result of eating too much meat, dairy food, and other animal protein that leech calcium and other minerals from the bones, as well as excessive salt, caffeine, alcohol, and smoking. In addition to avoiding or reducing these foods, natto is particularly effective in treating this affliction. Natto, fermented soybeans that clump together with long sticky strands, has been a staple in Far Eastern cooking and macrobiotic healthcare. It is especially beneficial for the intestines and digestion.

☤ Natto Helps Relieve Osteoporosis

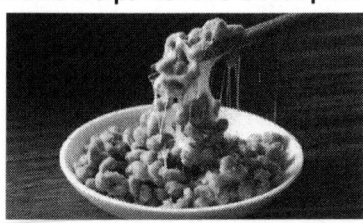

Natto, fermented soybeans, protect against bone loss

In a study on the effect of consuming natto on bone density, Japanese scientists found that total hipbone mineral density increased with increasing habitual natto intake in postmenopausal women, although not at other skeletal sites. There was also improvement at the fe-

femoral neck and at the radius in older women.[152] Natto's antibiotic and antitumor properties are now being investigated. It is also effective in reducing the effects of hangovers.

Pregnancy and Child Birth

The Kushis had five children, wrote *Raising Healthy Kids* and *Macrobiotic Pregnancy and Care of the Newborn* with Edward and Wendy Esko, longtime macrobiotic teachers and parents of eight children, and gave many seminars on children's and family health. As a rule, they recommended natural home birth or assistance of a midwife in a hospital setting. In many cases, dietary modification or adjustment would successfully deal with any problems encountered. However, for difficult deliveries, they sometimes recommended acupuncture, moxibustion (burning herbs to stimulate acupuncture points), or shiatsu massage. Prayer and meditation are also important healing methods they encouraged. At the Kushi Institute, the One Peaceful World Children's Shrine and Memorial was erected to honor the spirits of unborn children who died prematurely through abortion, miscarriage, accident, or disease. Modern medicine has validated the use of traditional Far Eastern methods for assisting childbirth.

☥ Moxibustion Aids Breech Births

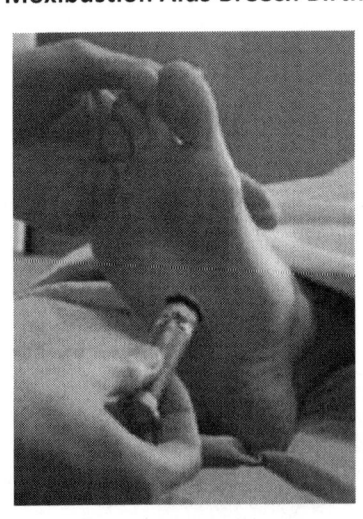

Moxa, or burning an herb on an acupressure point is effective for difficulty deliveries and many other conditions

In China, moxibustion (burning herbs to stimulate acupuncture points) was traditionally used to treat breech babies. In a study designed to evaluate the efficacy and safety of moxa, researchers at the Women's Hospital of Jiangxi Province, Nanchang, and Jiujiang Women's and Children's Hospital devised a clinical trial of 260 expectant mothers with breech presentation. The women were randomly divided into two groups. During the thirty-third week of pregnancy, the intervention group received stimulation of acupoint BL 67 (on the bladder meridian on the outside corner of the fifth toenail) for seven days with treatment for an additional seven days if necessary. Fetal movement correlated with overall success in righting the developing babies. The intervention group experienced an average of 48 fetal movements vs

35 in the control group and although 24 subjects in the control group and 1 in the intervention group underwent external cephalic version, 98 of the 130 fetuses in the intervention group were cephalic at birth vs 81 in the control group of 130 fetuses. The findings were published in the *Journal of the American Medical Association* and lauded by the AMA.[153]

☤ Moxa and Acupuncture May Reduce Caesarean Section

In a review of six trials of the traditional Chinese use of moxa for breech deliveries, researchers concluded, "There is some evidence to suggest that the use of moxibustion may reduce the need for oxytocin. When combined with acupuncture, moxibustion may result in fewer births by caesarean section; and when combined with postural management techniques may reduce the number of non-cephalic presentations at birth."[154]

☤ Shiatsu and Acupuncture Aid Childbirth

According to Chinese medicine, a correct balance of Qi (life energy) and quantity of blood are vital in order to commence labor and continue the childbirth process. Correspondingly, there are two main reasons for a delayed or difficult childbirth: lack of Qi and blood or stagnation of Qi and blood. In a retrospective study of 80 women aged 22-40 who required labor inducement, researchers compared traditional inducement methods (including shiatsu and/or acupuncture), conventional methods (pharmaceutical, mechanical), and a combination of both. Researchers

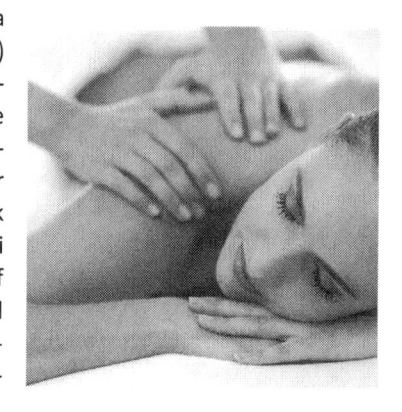

Shiatsu massage is relaxing and stimulates Ki energy flow

found that traditional inducement methods, whether or not combined with conventional methods, are an important and effective tool in their ability to reduce the extent of intervention throughout the birth process and also in reducing delivery completion interventions. "Significant difference was found in shortening labor process when inducement treatment combined both Chinese medicine and conventional methods, in comparison to conventional inducement alone {medicinal/mechanical)," the researchers concluded. "This is an important result considering the high availability and low cost of Chinese treatment, and especially because it is a non-harmful method of inducement."[155]

Lifestyle

Chewing

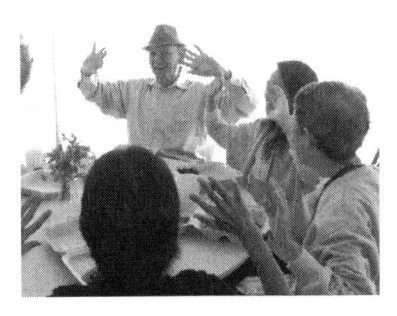

Thorough chewing benefits mind, body, and spirit. In a review of chewing and its effects, including many scientific and medical studies and personal accounts, two macrobiotic teachers and counselors conclude that proper chewing (approximately 50 or more times per mouthful) contributes to health at many levels:

Marathon chewer Lino Stanchich
leads a lunchtime discussion

- **Proper Digestion** Chewing protects against hunger, starvation, and disease and is essential for proper digestion; contributes to health and vitality, and prolongs life. It charges the food, activating the entire organism
- **Improves Taste of Food** Chewing improves the sensory qualities of food. It makes grains sweeter to the taste, stimulates the appetite, and contributes to greater awareness of texture, smell, and aroma
- **Stabilizes the Emotions** Chewing helps stabilize the emotions and by slowing down consumption and improving taste contributes to the aesthetic enjoyment of the meal
- **Calms the Mind** Chewing calms the mind, strengthens the intellect, and contributes to greater clarity, insight, and understanding
- **Reduces Food Waste** Chewing contributes to greater harmony within the family, in society, and with the environment, including better communication with others, increased awareness of earth and sky, and less use of energy and waste of food (including packaging materials, transport, and disposal)
- **Enhances Spiritual Awareness** Chewing contributes to spiritual awareness, including deeper knowledge of the order of nature and the universe, stronger intuition, and discovery of one's dream in life
- **Contributes to Universal Consciousness** Chewing contributes to universal awareness, including the free play of consciousness on all levels and oneness with all of life

In addition to examining the physiology of digestion, the study describes the traditional use of saliva for healing, especially by Jesus and Mohammad.[156]

Exercise and Fitness

Exercise, fitness, and physical activity are an important dimension of daily health. Eating a balanced, grain-centered diet can also translated into winning on the ball field.

Macrobiotic Japanese Baseball Team Wins Championship

In 1983, a Japanese professional baseball team climbed from last to first place by switching to a macrobiotic diet. After taking over the last place Seibu Lions in October, 1981, manager Tatsuro Hirooka initiated a dietary experiment. Restricting the players' intake of meat, sugar, and white rice, he encouraged them to eat brown rice, tofu, vegetables, and soybean products. He told the players that animal food increases an athlete's susceptibility to injuries. Conversely, natral foods, they were told, protect the body from sprains and dislocations and keep the mind clear and focused. During the 1982 season, the Lions were ridiculed by their archrivals, the Nippon Ham Fighters, a team sponsored by a major meat company. However, the Lions defeated the Ham-Fighters for the Pacific League crown and continued to the Japan World Series and beat the Chunichi Dragons. The Lions won the championship again the following year as well.[157]

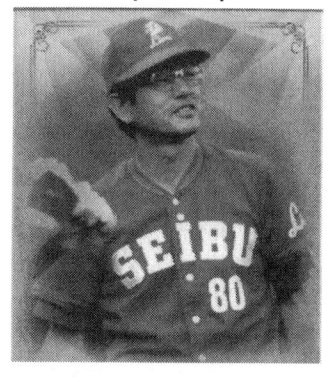

The Seibu Lions climbed from last to first place on a macrobiotic diet and defeated the Ham-Fighters

Arts and Culture

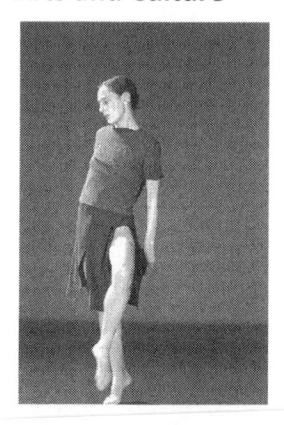

Many singers, dancers, and movie stars have observed a macrobiotic way or employed macrobiotic chefs, including Gloria Swanson, Maurice Cunningham, Madonna, Sting, Anne Teresa de Keeermacher, Demi Moore, Pamela Anderson, Gwyneth Paltrow, Alicia Silverstone, Fiona Apple, Nicole Kidman, Tom Cruise, and John Travolta. As singer John Denver enthused, "On a macrobiotic diet, I had all the energy in the world, clear-headed and singing like a bird! I loved it, I felt great!" In addition to a healthy glow, improved vitality, a trimmer physique, and greater flexibility, some performers also use macrobiotic principles:

Dancer Anne Teresa de Keersmacher

- **Composer John Cage** John Cage whom *Time* hailed as "the puckish composer, audacious theoretician, stylish writer, subtle graphic artist, macrobiotic guru and fearless mushroom hunter . . . the impish personification of the 20th century avant-garde" used the I Ching and Far Eastern principles to compose music. His colleague dancer Maurice Cunningham was also macrobiotic.[158]
- **Artist Rod House** Rod House, one of Michio Kushi's earliest students, taught at the New England College of Art, and was on the original faculty of the Kushi Institute. His paintings have been exhibited throughout New England.
- **Painter and Sculptor Patricia Price** Patricia Price, an English artist and painter, taught art at the Kushi Institute and sculpted a large Jizo Bodhisattva.
- **Dancer and Choreographer Anne Teresa de Keersmacher** Founder, director, and choreographer of Rosas Dance Company in Brussels, Anne Teresa uses yin and yang, the five transformations, and other macrobiotic principles in her compositions. Her company performs worldwide, e.g., staging spiral dances at the Museum of Modern Art (MoMA) in New York, and her dance school has a macrobiotic dining room.

Social Health

Ancient Food Pattern
Since the time of Darwin and the introduction of evolutionary theory, scientists believed that meat eating was largely responsible for the development of human prowess, intellect, and ingenuity. Over the last generation, a revolution in anthropology, archaeology, and other social sciences has led to an emerging view that ancient hominins were not primarily hunters, but gatherers, and that plant-based foods largely shaped and influenced our unique human qualities.

- **Present Day Hunter-Gatherers Eat Mostly Plants**
  Contemporary hunter-gather societies such as the Son and Kalahari bushmen in Africa consume the vast majority of their food in the form of foraged plants, fruits, and nuts and only small amounts, 10-20%, in the form of animal food.[159]

- **Evidence of Plant-Based Diets Doesn't Survive Well**
  "The archaeological evidence [for plant-eating] is especially weak, as many organic materials, especially plants, do not survive well, and are therefore invisible in the archaeological record," the *European Journal of Clinical Nutrition* reported in 2002. Artifacts, such as stone tools which are likely to be used for hunting and animal bones with evidence of hu-

man processing and butchering do indicate that hunting did occur at many times in the past, but it is impossible to judge the frequency."[160]

⚕ Cooking Made Us Human

In *Catching Fire: How Cooking Made Us Human,* Harvard primatologist Richard Wrangham hypothesized that the mastery of fire for cooking spurred the development of early humans, not meat-eating. Cooking, in his view, made more calories from existing, largely plant quality foods, available and improved metabolism, leading to the development of larger brains. Cooking also facilitated warmth, leading to the loss of body hair and the ability to run faster without overheating. Wrangham suggests it also allowed early hominins to develop more peaceful personalities, develop new social structures around the hearth, and bring the sexes closer together. Raw food, he contends, does not supply enough caloric energy and is unsustainable and can cause up to half the women to cease menstruation. Cooking increases the net energy gain by 30%.[161] As humans evolved from the monkey and primate state, they discovered cycles of change, found ways to store food, and learned to cook. As a result of his investigations, Wrangham became vegetarian.

⚕ Wild Grasses as Principal Food

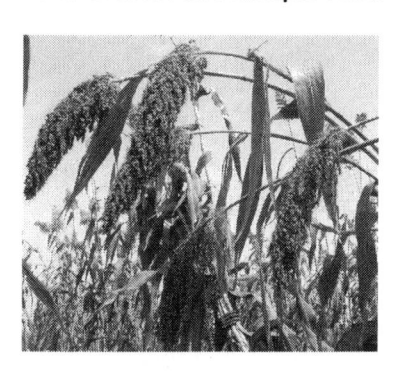

Sorghum appears to be ancient humans ancestral grain in Africa

In the early twenty-first century, evidence started to emerge that *homo sapiens* ate wild grasses, the prototype of grains, as principal food. At the University of Colorado Boulder researchers reported: "High tech tests on tooth enamel by researchers indicate that prior to about 4 million year ago, Africa's hominids were eating essentially chimpanzee style, dining on fruits and some leaves," explained anthropology professor Matt Sponheimer, lead author of the 2013 study. "A new look at the diets of ancient African hominids shows a 'game change' occurred about 3.5 million years ago when some members added grasses or sedges (a family of rushes including water chestnut) to their menus."[162] "It is quite possible that these changes in diet were an important step in becoming human," he concluded.

⚕ Lucy, Mother of Humankind, a Vegetarian

For nearly 2 million years, *Australopithecus,* the primary hominin ancestors in Africa, was largely vegetarian. *Australopithecus anamensis*, a hominid that lived in East Africa more than 4 millions years ago, was herbivorous. Lucy, often referred to as the Eve or mother of the human race, lived about a million years later. Her skeletal remains, found in East Africa, classify her as *Australopithecus afarensis*. She was vegetarian, eating grasses and leaves, as well as fruit, nuts, seeds, and tubers.[163]

⚕ Homo Sapiens Harvested Wild Grains

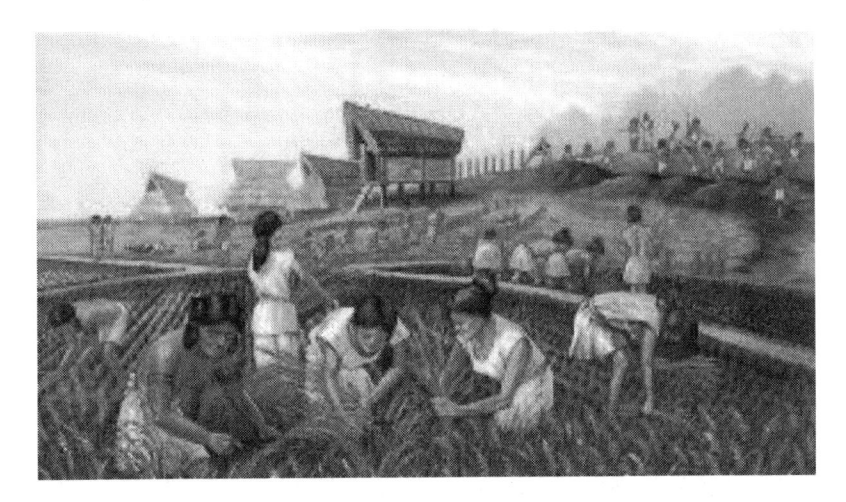

Homo sapiens **have been harvesting wild grain, processing, and consuming it for at least half of its existence**

Stone tools recently found in East Africa, the cradle of humanity, showed that people were processing sorghum 100,000 years ago. In Ngalue, a cave in Mozambique, researchers discovered an assortment of seventy stone tools in a layer of sediment deposited on the cave floor 42,000 to 105,000 years ago. Although the tools cannot be dated precisely, those in the deepest strata appear to be at least 100,000 years old. About 80% of the tools, including scrapers, grinders, points, flakes, and drills, had ample starchy residue, archaeologists told *Science*.[164] Eighty-nine percent of the starches came from sorghum, a cereal grain that still constitutes a main staple in many parts of Africa. The rest came from the African wine palm, the false banana, pigeon peas, wild oranges, and the African potato. The evidence suggests that people living in Ngalue routinely brought starchy plants, especially sorghum, to their cave where it was made into porridge and baked in the form of flat bread.

⚕ Prehistoric European Bakeries

In multiple European sites, including present-day Moravia, Italy, and Russia, evidence has surfaced of ancient grain harvesting, cooking, and processing dating to about 25,000 to 30,000 years ago, a Stone Age era renowned for its elegant Ice Age cave paintings. For example, mammoth hunters in Dolni Vestonice, an Upper Paleolithic site in Moravia, had sickle blades and grinding stones. Researchers speculate that they harvested edible seeds of wild grasses, the common reed, bog bean, water nut, and arctic berries.[165] Remains of plant food preserved by a hearth at Dolni Vestonice II dating to from 27,000 to 24,000 years ago contained a seed, tissues from roots and tubers, possible acorn mush, and wood charcoal. In the Black Sea region, archaeologists unearthed thousands of small blades made of flint and hafted with bitumen into bone handles to harvest wild grasses and cane. As Dr Revedin of the Italian Institute of Prehistory and Early History in Florence concluded: "The discovery of grain and plant residues on grinding stones at the three sites suggests plant-based food processing, and possibly flour production, was common and widespread across Europe at least 30,000 years ago."[166]

Food and Agriculture

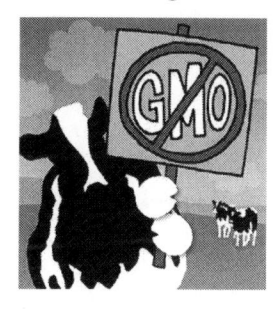

The macrobiotic community mobilized to protect rice, wheat, and other key foods from genetic engineering

The introduction of genetically engineered foods in the 1990s fundamentally altered the human food supply. The Sacramento Valley in northern California is the site of most of the organic brown rice production in the United States. In 2000, Monsanto announced plans to introduce GMO rice in the region, a step that would almost certainly have resulted in the contamination of organic rice and the main staple in the macrobiotic community. Macrobiotic teachers Alex Jack, Edward Esko, Bettina Zumdick, and their associates formed Amberwaves, a grassroots network to educate the public about the potential dangers of genetically engineered crops. The campaign included a petition that garnered tens of thousands of signatures, concerts known as Amberfests, workshops and lectures, books and articles, and meetings with the California Rice Commission, FDA, EPA, and members of Congress. In the end, Monsanto was defeated, and GMO rice was never commercialized in the United States or elsewhere in the world. Amberwaves also helped prevented Monsanto from introducing GMO wheat.[167]

☤ GMO Foods Imperil Natural Evolution

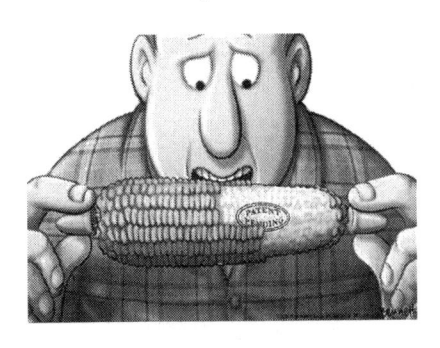

In a review of more than 100 scientific and medical studies on genetically engineered seeds, crops, and foods, an Amberwaves researcher concluded that GMOs pose a serious threat to continued natural biological and spiritual evolution. "Even before genetic engineering was developed, an estimated 97 percent of all native species of grains, beans, vegetables, and fruits in America disappeared in the 20th century, driven to extinction by monoculture, hybrid seeds, jet transportation, and modern economies of scale . . . It will take dramatic concerted action to protect freedom of choice, end the war on nature, and ensure the health of American and the planet as a whole."[168]

An estimated 70% of all processed foods in US supermarkets contain GMO corn, soy, or cotton

☤ GMO Rice Harmful to Human Health

LibertyLink Rice, the first GMO rice developed in America, was grown experimentally in Texas in 2001. Amberwaves commissioned Joe Cummins, a Canadian geneticist who has written more than 200 research papers, to prepare a scientific report on LibertyLink Rice and its possible effects on human health and the environment. LL Rice is spliced with a gene that is resistant to glufosinate, an extremely toxic herbicide. In his study, Cummins reported that LibertyLink Rice would probably result in major adverse health effects to consumers and farmers, as well as reduced yields and the contamination of other plants.

"Glufosinate is a herbicide that kills almost everything green; it is used extensively with genetically engineered crops including corn, canola, and soybeans," he explained. "The herbicide resistant crops were approved by the Canadian and United States governments, even though there was clear evidence that the herbicide caused birth defects in experimental animals. The chemical acts by causing premature cell death in the immature brain by a process called apotosis. It also prevents development of glutamate channels in the brain, thus disrupting cellular communication. The birth defects observed in animals included brain defects leading to behavioral changes. Cleft lip and skeletal defects or kidney and urethra injury were observed in treated newborn. The herbicide also caused miscarriage and reduced conception in treated mothers. Exposure of male farm workers caused birth defects in their children."

As a result of a public campaign against GMO foods and the contamination of much of the nation's corn crop by an unapproved variety of modified corn, Aventis destroyed all 5 million pounds of LL Rice grown in Texas. Since then, there has been no commercialization of GMO rice.[169]

Crime and Violence

Food affects mood as well as physical health. Macrobiotic food has figured prominently in several prison projects and helped reduce crime and violence.

℞ Sugar Linked to Violent Behavior

Frank Kern, assistant director at Tidewater Detention Center in Chesapeake, Virginia, a state facility for juvenile offenders, initiated a double-blind dietary study. In 1979, Kern, a graduate of the Kushi Institute, arranged an experiment in which sugar was taken out of the meals and snacks of 24 inmates. Researchers found that the youngsters on the modified diet exhibited a 45 percent lower incidence of formal disciplinary actions and antisocial behavior than the control group. Follow-up studies showed that after limiting sugar there was an 82 percent reduction in assaults, 77 percent reduction in thefts, 65 percent reduction in horseplay, and 55 percent reduction in not obeying orders. The researchers also found that "the people most likely to show improvement were those who had committed violent acts on the outside." The findings appeared in *International Journal of Biosocial Research.*[170]

℞ Portuguese Prisoners Go Macrobiotic

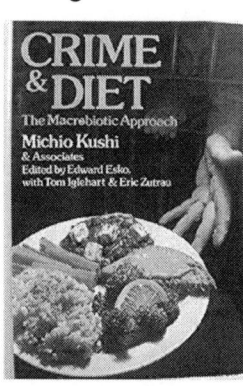

In prison, many inmates started macrobiotics and became peaceful and went on to productive lives

In 1979 several inmates at the Central Prison in Linho, a maximum security facility, outside of Lisbon, Portugal, began eating a macrobiotic diet and attending lectures on Oriental philosophy and medicine. Soon 30 prisoners had become macrobiotic, including Toze Areal, the leader of a bank robber gang, and prison officials allowed them to use a large kitchen where they cooked and ate together several times a week. As a result of attitude and behavioral changes, most of the prisoners attending classes received commutations and were released early. "[T]here is a great difference in them, especially in those who have left the prison," Senhor Alfonso, a prison administrator, noted, commenting on the macrobiotic group. "It is not easy to describe—for one thing I can say that now they take more initiative. Actually, there is no problem here with anyone who is macrobiotic; this way of life enjoys a very good reputation. I believe the food and the outside stimulus both helped. The food can change people." Areal went on to study at the Kushi Institute, marry and have a large family, and start a company that made tofu and tempeh.[171]

☤ GMOs Linked to Sexual Decline and School Violence

In a review of scientific and medical studies on GMOs, Alex Jack concluded that genetic engineering is contributing to abnormal sexual development, increased problems with conception, diminished sexual desire and performance, sex reversals and altered sex ratios, sterility, and other reproductive ills. He also examined the energetic effects of eating food produced from strains of GMO seeds developed with a gene gun—a pistol shooting modified .22 and .45 bullets coated with genetic material into the plant—and correlated the introduction of GMO foods with the increase of violence in society, especially among children and the dramatic increase in shootings and other violent incidents in schools.[172]

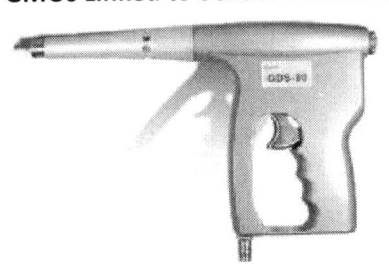

There may be a link between the outbreak of school shootings and consumption of GMO food strains created by the gene gun

Peace and Social Justice

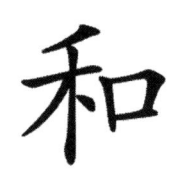

The Far Eastern word for peace is *wa* and is made up of two characters, or ideograms, for "grain" and "mouth." By eating a balanced whole grain diet, humans become calm and peaceful, see clearly, and exercise sound judgment. The Prophet Isaiah's dictum to turn swords into plowshares points at the same truth: peace comes from cultivating grains and eating in a plant-based way. Macrobiotic initiatives in the Middle East, South America, and other regions have helped reduce religious, ethnic, and class tensions and restore balance and harmony.

☪ Macrobiotic Food Unifies Warring Religions in Lebanon

Susana Sarué left the Sorbonne in Paris where she was completing her doctorate in nutrition to travel to the Middle East and used macrobiotic food and principles to help restore peace between warring Christians and Moslems in Beirut, as well as Palestinian refugees caught in the fighting, and Israeli soldiers and officials. She learned that there used to be a whole grain bread in Lebanon called Wise Bread because it gave wisdom, or nourishment, but for many years the bread had been made entirely with white flour. This flat bread composed about two-thirds of the daily diet. With donations, she and other macrobiotic practitioners opened a small bakery and brought the bread to the homes of many families who had a lot of children and who didn't have any work. Gradually people learned how to make the bread themselves. Later, a natural foods cooperative was set up and made grains, beans, miso, soy sauce, and other healthy foods available. In East Beirut,

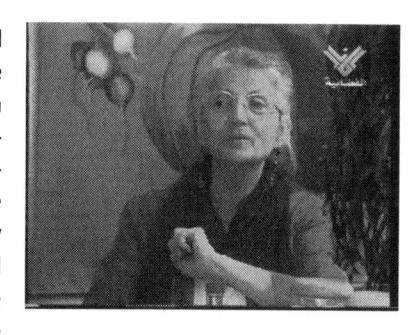

Miriam Nour, known as the Oprah of the Middle East, spreads macrobiotics through her daily TV show

Miriam Nour, a prominent journalist, began to work in the villages and eventually became the leading macrobiotic teacher after Susana returned home. "Other countries—America, France—send us donations: canned food, sugar, white flour, margarine," Nour observed. "And they send us free medication. It's a vicious circle—the food is eaten, the people get sick, they go to hospitals, they take the medications. The food is eaten, the people become more aggressive, angry, and warlike. And the people who send this junk food and medication, the synthetic clothing, also send the bombs. It is also they who say they want to make peace. But the war itself wants to fight because there is war in our hearts and minds." Nour went on to host the leading TV talk show in the Middle East and introduced macrobiotics to millions of people, including the leaders of many Islamic countries.[173]

Sugarcane Workers Gain Reforms after Dietary Change

In Virareka, a small village in Colombia, a sugarcane plantation had displaced local farms and fields. Over the years, large amounts of chemicals were applied to the cane, which came to displace all other crops. Deserts replaced green fields of grains and vegetables. Almost all the food eaten locally was brought in and consisted mainly of white flour, sugar, dairy food, meat, and other highly processed foods. Nutritionist Susana Sarué, a native of Latin America, returned to Colombia in the 1970s and developed a whole range of foods made from natural ingredients. She introduced a variety of cutlets, burgers, and other "meats" with a soya base, offered the people soy milk instead of dairy, and made an ice cream from sorghum and soya. The children's condition began to improve quickly. They became more alert and intelligent in school and less famished. They no longer had large stomachs. They also became more active. A health food bar was opened and managed by the local people. One day, the men of the village went on strike, and the bosses at the sugar plantation refused their demands, reasoning that they would starve after the third day and return to work. But the strikers, subsisting on local grains and beans and soy products, continued for two weeks, and the company was forced to give in and raise their wages.[174]

Teaching Macrobiotics in War-Torn Syria

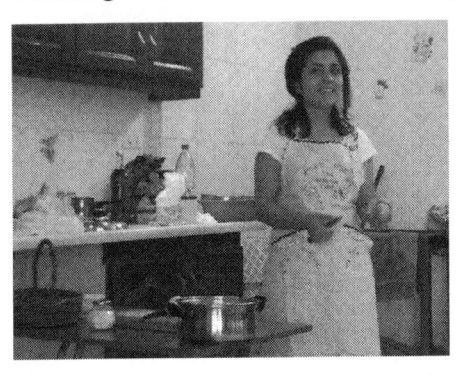

As the war in Syria spread, America and Russia initiated air strikes, and millions of refugees fled the country, Baydaa Laylaa, an elementary schoolteacher from Latakia, was busy giving macrobiotic cooking classes. Because of the war, the price of meat increased and people reduced their consumption. Because of sanctions, pharmacies are offering whole foods and herbal remedies instead of drugs. Sanctions have also reduced the availability of macrobiotic specialty foods. Fighting has disrupted organic farming, so vegetables have been in short supply. After marrying Hussain Muhammad, another graduate of the Kushi Institute in America, Baydaa moved to Kuwait with her husband, but the couple still returns to Syria periodically to teach and give health consultations. In the future, they would like to start an organic farm. "There is no organic farming now," she noted. "Organic produce is imported, but it is expensive and the Ki energy is depleted. We also want to start a macrobiotic kitchen and introduce a healthier way of eating to children, parents, and the general public."[175]

Baydda Laylaa gives cooking classes during the conflict in her country

Trauma Teams Aid Children in Asia

Through Fortunate Blessings Foundation, Bill and Joan Spear, macrobiotic teachers in Litchfield, Connecticut, began an international relief program in 2004 to assist children who had been traumatized from natural disasters, war, torture, and other misfortune. After the initial emergency phase of a disaster, Second Response Trauma Teams, staffed by mental health professionals, travel to the impacted area to offer emotional support. During PLAYshops, participants directly engage in an experiential session on methodologies that employ body or somatic exercises to release repressed emotions. In recent years, trauma teams have assisted children in Sri Lanka and Indonesia following the great tsunami, as well as victims of the Nepalese earthquake and the nuclear accident at Fukushima in Japan.[176]

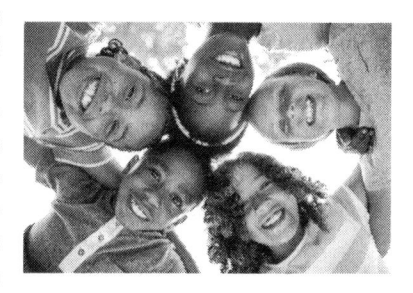

Second Response aids children following natural disasters, war, and nuclear accidents

Planetary Health

The macrobiotic way of eating is beneficial for the planet as well as personal and social health. It helps protect the soil, air, water, and other natural resources from artificial fertilizers, pesticides, and other chemicals. It respects the diversity of species and contributes to the flourishing of bees, butterflies, and other pollinators. It reduces greenhouse gases in the atmosphere and mitigates climate change. Conversely, the modern way of farming and eating is a main cause of global warming, climate change, and other environmental destruction.

Nutrient Decline

☤ Nutrients in Produce Decline 25 to 50 Percent

In an analysis of the latest U.S. Department of Agriculture food composition tables, macrobiotic researcher Alex Jack reported a sharp decline in minerals, vitamins, and other nutrients in many chemically grown common foods between 1997 and 1975 when the last comprehensive survey was published. A random sampling of twelve garden vegetables found that calcium levels declined on average 26.5 percent, vitamin A dropped 21.4 percent, and vitamin C fell 29.9 percent. Whole grains and beans also showed sharp fluctuations. The amount of calcium and iron in millet fell 60 percent and 55.7 percent, and thiamin and riboflavin declined 42.3 percent and 23.7 percent, but niacin rose 105.2 percent. Brown rice also showed mixed results, with slight decreases in calcium and riboflavin, and mild increases in iron, thiamine, and niacin. Overall, green leafy vegetables appeared to have lost the most nutrients, while root vegetables, beans, and grains lost the least. "Decline of the natural environment appears to be the major reason for the widespread loss of nutrients. . . . This suggests a steady deterioration in soil, air, and water quality, as well as reduced seed vitality, that is depleting minerals and other inorganic components of food," the study concluded. Following an Open Letter to the U.S. Secretary of Agriculture by the editors of *Organic Gardening*, the USDA verified the accuracy of the study, and it was confirmed by other researchers.[177]

Global Warming

☤ Modern Diet Main Cause of Global Warming

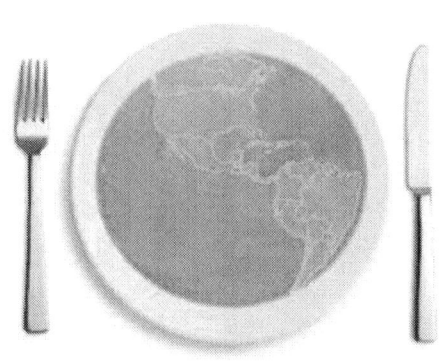

Livestock's Long Shadow, the landmark report of the United Nations' Food and Agricultural Organization (FAO) concluded, the modern food pattern is the key to preventing global warming, climate change, and other environmental destruction. The study found that the cattle and other livestock industries are the single biggest contributor to global warming, "responsible for 18% of greenhouse gas emissions measured by CO2 equivalent. This is a higher share than transport," or 40 percent more than all the cars, trucks, buses, trains, and planes combined. The meat industry is "one of the . . . most significant contributors to the most serious environmental problems, at every scale from local to global," including "problems of land degradation, climate change and air pollution, water shortage and water pollution, and loss of biodiversity." Global meat and milk consumption is expected to double by 2050, further accelerating environmental destruction and global warming.[178]

According to the United Nations, the modern food and agricultural system is the biggest contributor to climate change

☤ Dietary Change Saves More CO2 Than Buying a Prius

A 2006 study by Gidon Eishel and Pamela Martin at the University of Chicago found that a vegetarian diet is more energy efficient than one containing meat. The authors gathered data from many sources, examining the amount of fossil fuel energy required to sustain several different diets. The vegetarian diet turned out to be the most energy efficient, followed by a poultry-based diet and the standard American diet high in red meat. The authors compared a Toyota Prius, which uses about a quarter as much as fuel as a Chevrolet Suburban SUV, to a plant-based diet, which uses roughly one-fourth as much energy as a diet rich in red meat. Changing from a diet rich in red meat to a plant-based diet cuts greenhouse gas emissions as much as shifting from a Suburban SUV to a Prius.[179]

Global Warming Alters Food Composition

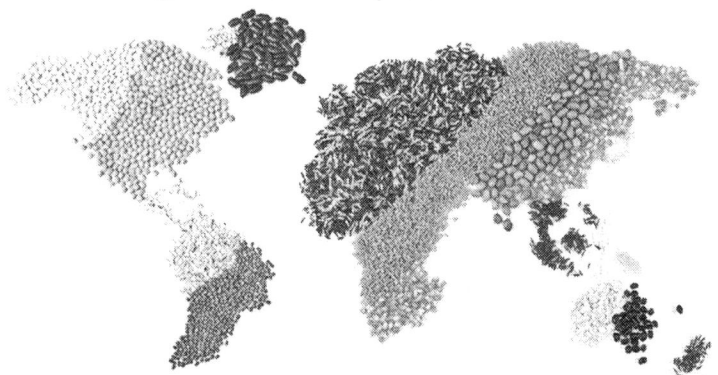

Global warming is dramatically altering the nutritional value of foods worldwide. As a result of rising CO2 levels in the atmosphere, protein and nitrogen concentrations are down up to 25 percent in wheat, rice, and other major staples, mineral and trace element content have fallen 8 percent on average in 130 common crops, and carbohydrate has soared from 10 to 45 percent, according to the first ecological study of its kind. The dramatic increase in starch and sugar content may be the main cause of "hidden hunger" and the global obesity epidemic.

Elevated CO2 levels have reduced the overall concentration of 25 important minerals, including calcium, iron, potassium, and zinc, in plants by an average of 8 percent. The reduction in the nutritional value of crops could have profound impacts on human health. A mineral-deficient diet can cause malnutrition, even if a person consumes adequate calories. This pattern of eating is common in developing countries because most people eat a limited number of staples. Diets low in minerals, especially iron and zinc, lead to reduced growth in childhood, to reduced natural immunity and protection from infection, and higher rates of maternal and child deaths and sickness.

The study suggests that the altered nutrient profiles are contributing to the rise in obesity, as people eat too many high starch foods to begin with, and now as the earth warms these foods are increasing their proportion of simple sugars. Consumers also eat more to compensate for the lower mineral content in other foods. "The new evidence supports an emerging view that while obesity is quantified as an imbalance between energy inputs and expenditures, it could also be a form of malnutrition, where increased carbohydrate:protein and excessive carbohydrate consumption could be possible targets," observed Irakli Loladze, a mathematical biologist and quantitative ecologist, at the University of Maryland University College.

The study acknowledges that mineral declines in crops may be a consequence of the Green Revolution that relied on increased amounts of pesticides and artificial fertilizers that depleted the soil and altered mineral content.[180]

Electromagnetic Fields

The electronics and digital revolution has bathed the planet in artificial electromagnetic radiation from satellites, televisions, cell phones, computers, tablets, smart meters, and other devices known as the Internet of Things. The long-term effects on human health and the environment are unknown. However, short-term studies have linked cell phones to brain tumors and disruption of glucose metabolism. They also disrupt wildlife, including the navigation systems of bees, butterflies, and other pollinators that are crucial to the world food supply.

⚕ Mobile Phones Disrupt Bees

Germany scientists reported that the electromagnetic radiation emitted by mobile phones and base stations can interfere with the bees' navigation systems, rendering them unable to find their way back to their hives. In an experiment conducted by researchers at Landau University, bees refused to return to a hive when a mobile phone was placed nearby. Although not conclusive, the experiment offers one possible explanation for the mysterious worldwide decline in the bee population known as Colony Collapse Disorder (CCD). Other factors, including pesticides, the varroa mite, viruses, genetically modified crops, and unusually cold winters, are also believed to contribute to the decline.[181]

⚕ Cell Phones Linked to Brain Tumors

In the most conclusive study to date linking non-ionizing cell phone radiation to brain cancer, research conducted by the National Toxicology Program (NTP) reported in 2016 that rats exposed to RF (radio frequency) radiation had higher rates of glioma (a type of brain tumor), as well as malignant schwannoma (a very rare heart tumor) than unexposed rates. Radiation exposure showed a direct dose-response relationship. Otis W. Brawley, M.D., chief medical officer for the American Cancer Society, stated: "The NTP report linking radiofrequency radiation (RFR) to two types of cancer marks a paradigm shift in our understanding of radiation and cancer risk."[182]

Energy and Transmutation

In 1959 French scientist Louis Kervran started publishing his discoveries in the field of biological transmutation—the synthesis of necessary, but unavailable, chemical elements out of simpler, available ones. He showed that in living biological systems sodium could change into potassium, manganese could be obtained from iron, silica from calcium, and phosphorus from sulfur. Macrobiotic educator George Ohsawa affirmed these findings, which flew in the face of conventional physics and chemistry. He had long taught that everything in the universe is subject to the law of change and that transmutation of elements at ordinary temperatures and pressures was possible. Critics dismissed this view as alchemy, contending that such transmutations could only occur under stellar or nuclear conditions. Michio Kushi assisted Ohsawa in several experiments verifying the process and went on to herald the discovery as the catalyst for a new industrial revolution. He predicted that it would eventually replace mining and its toll on human life and environmental destruction and make valuable resources commonly available for the betterment of society and a sustainable future.

☤ Saharan Workers Transmute Sodium to Potassium in Body

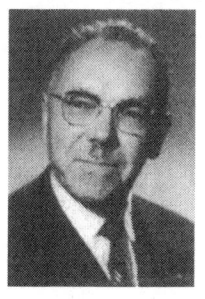

Louis Kervran, pioneer investigator of biological transmutation

In 1959 French scientist Louis Kervran started publishing his discoveries in the field of biological transmutation —the synthesis of necessary but unavailable chemical elements out of simpler, available ones. His interest in this field began when he studied workers in the Sahara desert, who excreted more sodium than they consumed. Tests showed a comparable amount of potassium was being taken. Kervran showed potassium was capable of being transmuted into sodium in the body. Developing the theories of George Ohsawa that elements can be transmuted into one another peacefully without smashing the atom, Kervran went on to find that iron could be made from manganese, silica from calcium, and phosphorus from sulfur. Kervran's experiments have wide industrial, scientific, and social applications. For example, biological transmutations could be applied to rendering harmless nuclear wastes, toxic spills, and other chronic environmental hazards.[183]

☤ Changing Carbon into Iron

Seeking to replicate Kervran's sodium to potassium experiment in the laboratory, George Ohsawa conducted a tabletop test in Tokyo in the early 1960s. Inserting positively and negatively charged electrodes into a vacuum tube, 2.3 mg of sodium combined with 1.6 mg of oxygen allowed to enter the tube and formed 3.9 mg of potassium. In another experiment, Ohsawa used a graphite crucible to transmute carbon into iron. He subsequently conducted other experiments until his death in 1966.[184]

☤ Pentagon Verifies Transmutation

U.S. military scientists tested the theory of biological transmutations and in 1978 verified the transmutation of matter from cell to cell and atom to atom. Surveying the works of Kervran and Ohsawa, researchers concluded "granted the existence of such transmutations (Na to Mg, K to Ca, and Mn to Fe), then a net surplus of energy was also produced. A proposed mechanism was described in which Mg adenosine triphosphate, located in the mitochondrion of the cell, played a double role as an energy producer. . . . The relatively available huge supplies of the elements which have been reported to have been transmuted and the probable large accompanying energy surplus indicate a new source of energy may be in the offing—one whose supply would be unlimited."[185]

☤ 20 Key Industrial Elements Created

Quantum Rabbit LLC, a small macrobiotic company based in Massachusetts, transmuted small amounts of elements in a series of experiments between 2005 and 2016. In carbon-arc studies based on the Ohsawa/Kushi model, the QR team, consisting of Edward Esko, Alex Jack, and Woodward Johnson, produced from pure graphite (carbon) iron, magnesium, aluminum, silicon, scandium, titanium, cobalt, and nickel. Neodymium magnets showed the presence of magnetic activity, and an independent laboratory confirmed the presence of the metals in treated samples. A series of vacuum tube studies on noble gases fused helium plasma with oxygen to produce trace amounts of argon. In alkali metal vapor tests under vacuum, the QR team was able to produce potassium, copper, tin, germanium, and other elements. The QR researchers were able to produce potassium, palladium, strontium, silver, and gold. Results of more than a dozen studies were published in *Infinite Energy*, a journal dedicated to clean new energy sources.[186]

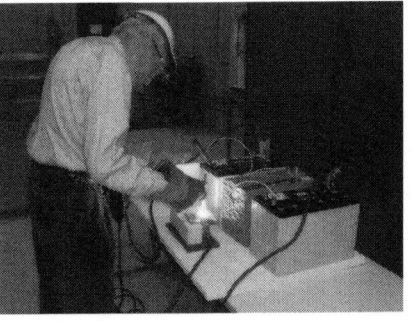

Woody Johnson conducting carbon arc studies for Quantum Rabbit

Light Pollution

☤ Dark Skies Vanishing

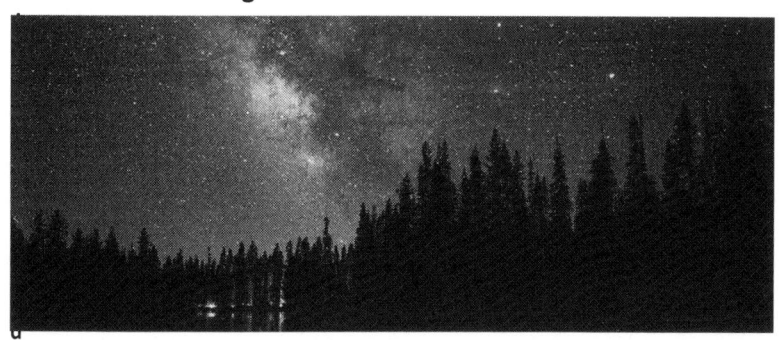

80% of the world lives under light-polluted skies and can't see the Milky Way

A new atlas of artificial night sky brightness shows that more than 80% of the world population and more than 99% of Americans, Europeans, and Japanese live under light-polluted skies.[187] Researchers report that the Milky Way is not visible to 80% of Americans and 60% of Europeans. This also includes Iraq, Syria, and other parts of the Middle East, where warfare has artificially lit up the sky.

Principal sources of light pollution are residential lights, streetlights, highway lights, motor vehicle headlights, sport stadium lights, electronic advertising billboards, shopping mall lights, park lights, airport lights, and offshore oil platforms.

The artificial light around cities and extending into many rural areas has interfered with the migration of nocturnal birds because they cannot follow the moon and stars. Light pollution also disorients bats, moths, and other animals that come out at night, and millions are killed each year by flying into streetlights. The metabolism of turtles, snakes, salamanders, and frogs has also been altered, as well as many plants.

Light pollution also affects humans, disrupting sleep, causing headaches, affecting sensory nerves, and contributing to depression. Alteration of circadian rhythms is further believed to increase the risk of obesity and diabetes. Some medical researchers suggest that artificial light, especially the blue component in white light at night, is carcinogenic.

From a macrobiotic perspective, the Milky Way and other stars shape and influence biological and spiritual evolution. As an article in *Amberwaves* noted: "They constantly charge our mid and forebrains, eyes, chakras, meridians, and other systems, organs, and functions, especially if we eat whole cereal grains that have awns or small antennae that receive and concentrate this cosmic energy and vibration. This current of incoming spiral energy orients us to beauty, truth, peace, justice, freedom, and other universal ideals. With the eclipse of night, the consciousness of modern society is rapidly dimming. . . .By respecting the natural rhythms and cycles of nature, including day and night, humanity can pass safely through this time. We can recover the compass of yin and yang, apply it to problems of society, and create a naturally bright new era."[188]

Controversies

As with any movement, the macrobiotic community has had its share of controversies. Debate has raged on many aspects of food quality. What is the best quality and amount of salt to use in cooking? Should rice and other grains be soaked prior to cooking and if so for how long? Should herbs and spices, if any, be consumed in a cold, northern climate? Is it better to eat food grown isn't organic?

Though most scientific and medical studies have found that the macrobiotic diet meets, and in many cases, exceeds current nutritional guidelines, the subject of Vitamin B-12 continues to spark controversy. Nutritionist T. Colin Campbell explains that B-12 originates naturally in the soil with microbes and is consumed in sufficient amounts by vegans who eat organic produce, especially that which is harvested and sold with some dirt clinging to the roots.

Cancer has also been a major topic of discussion. Despite many successful recoveries and studies showing that the macrobiotic approach can be effective, several teachers and counselors have come down with the disease, including the Kushis. Factors contributing to their illness (cervical and colon cancer respectively) included overwork, constant travel, irregular eating and eating out when abroad, lack of exercise, and taking on the energy and vibration of the many cancer patients with whom they worked. Both Aveline and Michio recovered from their initial diagnoses after a return to careful eating and lived for many more years (to age 78 and 88 respectively). Finding a balance among diet, lifestyle, and environmental factors is a constant challenge in today's modern world.

As conventional medicine has recognized the benefits of macrobiotics over the last half century, so macrobiotics has developed a respect for the use of surgery, drugs, and invasive treatments if diet and lifestyle approaches are not working. The trend toward integrative medicine, combining alternative and conventional therapies, is now widely supported in the macrobiotic community.

The Coming Era

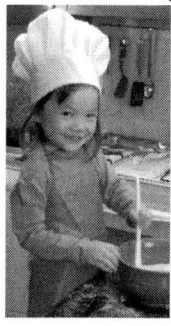

"The macrobiotic revolution is the most peaceful and effective way to restore the earth," as Michio Kushi observed. "Through it we are able to save ourselves and our families and friends from the vast current of degeneration sweeping the globe. We are even able to turn the general trend of modern civilization in a healthier, constructive direction. And, ultimately, we are able to enter the gateway of the new world, the Era of Humanity, with health and peace, justice and freedom, leading toward the unlimited happiness of all humanity for endless generations to come."[189]

Despite all the challenges, the macrobiotic community sees a bright, happy future for the planet and future generations

Appendix
On the Absolute Sincerity of Great Physicians

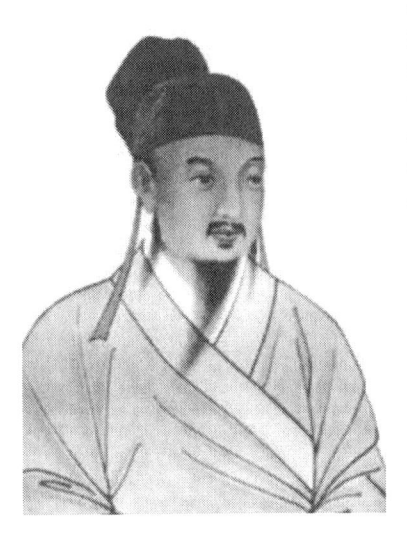

Sun Simiao, King of Medicine

Sun Simiao (581-682 CE), a Chinese medical pioneer during the Tang Dynasty composed several medical classics including Precious Prescriptions for Emergencies *and* On the Absolute Sincerity of Great Physicians, *a celebrated oath for physicians that came to be known as China's Hippocratic Oath:*

I promise to follow the way of the great physician. I will serve to live in harmony with nature, and teach patients to do the same.

I will stay calm and completely committed when treating disease. I will not give way to personal wishes and desires, but above all else hold and nurture a deep feeling of compassion.

I will be devoted to the task of saving the sacred spark of life in every creature that still carries it. I will strive to maintain a clear mind and be willing to hold myself to the highest standards.

It will be my duty to diagnose suffering and treat disease. I will not be boastful about my skills and not driven by greed for material things.

Above all, I will keep an open heart. As I move on the right path I will receive great happiness as a reward without asking for anything in return.

Macrobiotic Resources

Macrobiotic Education

Education has been the main focus of the modern macrobiotic community. The Ohsawas, Kushis, Aiharas, and other pioneers all saw themselves foremost as educators, introducing macrobiotic principles and practices to the general public as well as training students to become teachers, counselors, and cooks. Over the years, there have been many schools, centers, and events, including the Ohsawa Foundation, East West Foundation, Nippon C.I., Vega Institute, Community Health Foundation, Kushi Institute, and Holistic Cruise at Sea. Today the international macrobiotic network consists of hundreds of centers, mostly local and regional. Summer camps or conferences have been a feature of the movement for over a half-century, with annual get togethers at camps, hotels, colleges, and other venues around the world. Increasingly, classes, webinars, and video presentations are offered online and there are many macrobiotic oriented groups on Facebook and other social media.

Classes in theory and practice have formed the foundation of macrobiotic education. Schools and institutes typically offer a combination of lectures and hands on training, including certification, in the following:

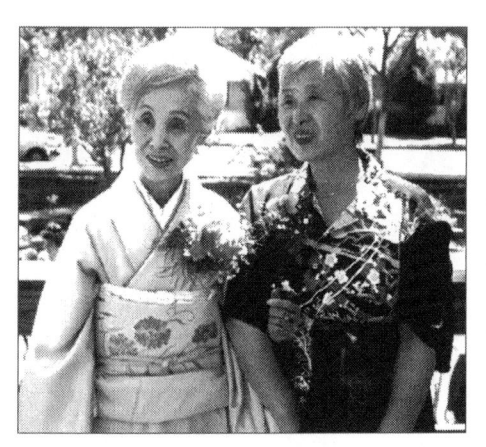

Lima Ohsawa and Shizuko Yamamoto, pioneer macrobiotic educators

- **Macrobiotic Philosophy** Studies and training in cosmology, philosophy, and science (often known as Order of the Universe), including the spiral of life, yin and yang, the five transformations, the four elements, biological evolution, man and woman, cycles of history, mythology and religion, agriculture and energy, transformation of society, transmutation of elements, the vibrational and spiritual world.

- **Macrobiotic Health Care** Studies and training in anatomy and physiology, the meridian and chakra system, origin and development of health and disease, classification of conditions by yin and yang and the five transformations, dietary guidelines and practice, macrobiotic nutrition, counselor training and practice

- **Macrobiotic Diagnosis** Studies and training in diagnosis and evaluation using sight, hearing, touch, taste, smell, and the other senses, as well as thoughts, emotions, dreams, visions, intuition, and other levels of consciousness; constitution and condition; Nine Star Ki and Oriental and Western Astrology, I Ching, and other metaphysical arts

- **Macrobiotic Cooking** Studies and training in daily cooking, seasonal cooking, gourmet and holiday cooking, travel food, medicinal cooking, restaurant cooking, catering, and other styles; home food production of miso, tofu, pickles, mochi, bread, and many other foods; menu planning; teacher and counselor training

- **Macrobiotic Energy Healing** Studies and training in shiatsu massage, do-in self-massage, stretching exercises, yoga, chanting, meditation, visualization, music and sound therapy, art and literature, and other disciplines

International Centers

- **Planetary Health, Inc.** A nonprofit educational organization in western Massachusetts founded and directed by Alex Jack, Edward Esko, Bettina Zumdick, and their associates, sponsoring the annual Macrobiotic Summer Conference and the Macrobiotic Wellness Retreat at Eastover, a holistic resort in Lenox, MA. Planetary Health, Inc., the parent nonprofit, also sponsors Amberwaves, a grassroots network to protect rice, wheat, and other grains from genetic engineering, climate change, and other challenges. Amberwaves Press publishes a quarterly journal and books and booklets. Contact: Box 487, Becket MA 01223, 413-623-0012. macrobioticwellnessretreat.com and macrobioticsummerconference.com.

- **George Ohsawa Macrobiotic Foundation** founded by Herman and Cornelia Aihara and now directed by Carl Ferre publishes the bimonthly *Macrobiotics Today* and books. GOMF, PO Box 3998, Chico, CA 95927. Tel: 530-566-9765. www.ohsawamacrobiotics.com. Email: gomf@earthlink.net

- **Fortunate Blessings Foundation**, nonprofit directed by William and Joan Spear, devoted to assisting children who have been traumatized from natural disasters, war, and torture. 409 Bantam Road, Suite A-3, Litchfield, CT 06759. (860) 567-8801. www.fortunateblessings.org.

- **Holistic Holiday at Sea**, an annual macrobiotic and holistic oriented cruise in the Caribbean founded by Sandy Pukel. 434 Aragon Ave, Coral

Gables, FL 33134, 305-725-0081, www.atasteofhealth.org. Email: info@holisticholidayatsea.com

- **Kushi Institute of Europe**. Co-founded and directed by Wieke Nelissen and Adelbert Nelissen (1949-2014). Weteringschans 65, 1017RX Amsterdam, The Netherlands. Tel: 011 31 20 625 7513. Website: www.macrobiotics.nl. Email: kushi@macrobiotics.nl

- **Kushi Macrobiotic School of Japan** in Tokyo founded and directed by Patricio Garcia de Parades. 3-14-16 Nishihara, Shibuya-ku, Tokyo 151-0066, Japan. Tel: +81-3-6326-6746. Website: www.kushischool.jp. Email: info@kushi-school.jp

- **Kushi School of the U.K.**, founded and directed by Nicola and David McCarthy. Offering programs south of London in conjunction with the Kushi Institute of Europe. 112 South Road, Haywards Heath, West Sussex, RH16 4 LL, UK. Tel: 01444 628667, www.kushischool.uk. Email: david@kushischool.uk

- **Macrobiotics America**, online institute founded and directed by David and Cynthia Briscoe from Oroville, California. 1735 Robinson St. #1874, Oroville, CA 95965, Tel: Tel: 530-521-0236. www.macroamerica.com. Email: info@macroamerica.com.

- **Sha Wellness Clinic**, a luxury spa on the Mediterranean Sea in Spain offering macrobiotic counseling, yoga, detox, and other personal services. 5 Verderol El Albir 03581 Alicante, Spain. +34 966 811 199. Website: shawellnessclinic.com. Email: info@shawellness.clinic.com.

- **Strengthening Health Institute,** founded and directed by Denny and Susan Waxman, offering online instruction from Philadelphia. 1940 S 10th St, Philadelphia, PA 19148, Tel: (215) 238-9212. www.strengtheninghealth.com.

- **Vegetarian Educational Institute**, sponsor of the annual Summer Retreat at Pinecrest Lake, California. Tel: (415) 226-9677. www.healthyhappyretreats.com. Email: info@healthyhappyretreats.com.

Macrobiotic Counseling

Personal dietary and way of life sessions are offered by many macrobiotic teachers and counselors in person, by Skype, over the phone, or by written report. While each practitioner has a slightly different approach, they generally include a review of the person's dietary and health history and background, visual diagnosis, specific dietary guidelines, way of life suggestions, and home remedies. Sessions take from about 1 to 1 ½ hours and cost from $200-$350. Modest follow up advice is included.

Macrobiotic Publishing

George Ohsawa healed himself after reading a book, and publishing has been an integral part of macrobiotics ever since. The Kushis and their associates composed several hundred books over the years, including basic texts on macrobiotic philosophy, health and healing, cooking, and shiatsu and do-in, as well as poetry, novels, art, literature, music, and other subjects. Principal publishers included the George Ohsawa Macrobiotic Foundation, Japan Publications, St. Martin's Press, One Peaceful World Press, Avery Publications, Square One Publications, Publicaciones Gea, and Amberwaves Press.

Macrobiotic Restaurants

Hundreds of macrobiotic restaurants, diners, snack bars, and take out kitchens have made delicious, healthful food available and influenced society at many levels. Major macrobiotic oriented restaurants today include: Inaka, M Café, Shojin (Los Angeles), Seed Kitchen (Venice CA), Paul & Elizabeth's (Northampton MA), Bizen (Great Barrington MA), Souen, Mana, Ozu, and Candle Cafe (NYC), Masao's Kitchen (Boston metro), Deshima (Amsterdam), Macrobiotic Zen Restaurant (Barcelona), Usagi Botanica (Morioka, Japan), Chaya (Tokyo), Las Casas (Austin TX), Wholly Macro (Palm Springs FL), Shangri-La Vegan (Oakland), .

Macrobiotic Food Companies

Pioneer macrobiotic food companies included Erewhon Trading Company, which the Kushis started in the mid-1960s and today is a division of General Mills; Chico-San, which Herman and Cornelia Aihara and other macrobiotic friends in northern California started and was incorporated into Quaker Oats; Lima Foods in Belgium, later purchased by a big company; Manna Foods, founded by Adelbert and Wieke Nelissen in Amsterdam; Muso and Mitoko, major macrobiotic food manufacturers in Japan; Clearspring, headed by Chris Dawkins in the UK; and many others. Key companies today include:

- **Eden Foods** a leading macrobiotic food manufacturer and distributor in the United States founded and directed by Michael Potter. Many of its products are available through mail order. Website: www.edenfoods.com

- **Gold Mine Natural Foods**, a macrobiotic distributor in San Diego, CA, specializes in heirloom grains, beans, and seeds. Website: www.goldminenaturalfoods.com.

- **Maine Coast Sea Vegetable Company** is a macrobiotic food company in Maine that harvests alaria (wakame), laver (nori), kelp, and other sea vegetables from the Atlantic Ocean. Website: www.seaveg.com

- **Maine Seaweed** is a macrobiotic-oriented sea vegetable company run by Larch Hanson. Website: www.theseaweedman.com

- **Natural Import Company**, a macrobiotic distributor in Asheville, NC. Website: www.naturalimport.com

- **Rhapsody** is a macrobiotic food company in Vermont that makes organic tempeh, miso amazake, *natto*, rice milk, vegan egg rolls, and other products. Website: www.rhapsodynaturalfoods.com

- **Si Sea Salt** is harvested from Pacific Ocean waters off the coast of Baja's Southern California. Website: www.sisalt.com

- **South River Miso**, a macrobiotic company in western Massachusetts, makes a variety of misos, including barley, brown rice, dandelion and leek, azuki bean, chickpea and millet. Website www.southrivermiso.com

Books and Literature

* = Highly recommended

Cookbooks
*Kushi, Aveline; Jack, Alex (1985). *Aveline Kushi's Guide to Macrobiotic Cooking for Health, Harmony, and Peace*. Warner Books. ISBN 0-446-38634-0.
Esko, Edward, and Wendy Esko (1981). *Macrobiotic Cooking for Everyone*. Japan Publications. ISBN 978-0870404696.
Esko, Wendy (1978). Aveline Kushi's *Introducing Macrobiotic Cooking*. Japan Publications, revised 1988. ISBN 978-0870406904.
Ferré, Julia (2007). *Basic Macrobiotic Cooking: 20th Anniversary Edition*. George Ohsawa Macrobiotic Foundation. ISBN 978-0918860590.
Jack, Alex; Jack, Gale (2000). *Amber Waves of Grain: Traditional American Whole Foods Cooking & Contemporary Vegetarian, Vegan & Macrobiotic Cuisine.*

One Peaceful World Press. ISBN 1-88294-37-4.

Jack, Alex; Kato, Sachi (2017). *The One Peaceful World Cookbook: Over 150 Vegan, Macrobiotic Recipes for Vibrant Health and Happiness,* BenBella. ISBN 978-1944648244.

Kushi, Aveline, with Wendy Esko (1984). *The Changing Seasons Macrobiotic Cookbook.* Avery Publishing Group, revised 2003. ISBN 978-1583331644.

Lechasseur, Eric; Suzuki, Sanae (2007). *Love Eric & Sanae: Seasonal Vegan Macrobiotic Cuisine.* Mugen, LLC. ISBN 978-0977293711.

Miyaji, Masao and Evelyne (2014). *The ABCs of Vegan Home Cooking.* Blurb. ISBN 978-1320146449.

Nishimura, Mayumi (2012). *Mayumi's Kitchen.* Kodansha. ISBN 978-1568364810.

Ohsawa, Lima (1984.). *Macrobiotic Cuisine.* Japan Publications. ISBN 978-0870406003.

Pirello, Christina (2007). *Cooking the Whole Foods Way.* HP Books. ISBN 978-1557885173

Tara-Watson, Marlene (2013). *Macrobiotics for All Seasons.* North Atlantic Books. ISBN 978-1583945582.

Turner, Christina (2002). *The Self-Healing Cookbook: Whole Foods to Balance Body, Mind, and Moods.* Earthtones.

Zumdick, Bettina (2012). *Authentic Foods.* ISBN 9781478327639.

Diet, Health, and Healing

*Kushi, Michio; Jack, Alex (2010). *The Cancer-Prevention Diet.* St. Martin's Press. ISBN 978-0-312-56106-2.

*Kushi, Michio; Jack, Alex (2002). *The Macrobiotic Path to Total Health*: Ballantine. ISBN 0-345-43987-2.

*Kushi, Michio (2007). *The Do-In Way: Gentle Exercises to Liberate the Body, Mind, and Spirit.* Square One Publications. ISBN 978-0-7570-0268-7.

*Kushi, Michio (2007). *Your Body Never Lies. Square One Publications.* ISBN 978-0-7570-0267-0.

*Kushi, Michio; Van Cauwenberge, Marc, M.D. (2014). *Macrobiotic Home Remedies.* Square One Publications. ISBN 978-0-7570-0269-4.

Aihara, Herman (1986). *Acid & Alkaline.* George Ohsawa Macrobiotic Foundation. ISBN 978-0918860446.

Akizuki, Tatsuichiro, M.D. (1981). *Nagasaki 1945*: *The First Full-Length Eyewitness Account of the Atomic Bomb Attack on Nagasaki.* Quartet Books. ISBN 978-0704333826

Andrus, Erik; Elwell, Christian; Rooney, Ben (2017). *The Rice Revolution: Growing*

Organic Rice in New England. Amberwaves Press. ISBN 9781544048772.

Brown, Simon (2007). *Modern-Day Macrobiotics*. North Atlantic Books. ISBN 978-1556436437.

Dufty, William (1975). *Sugar Blues*. Warner Books, 1986. ISBN 978-0446343121

Kushi, Michio (1987). *Crime & Diet: The Macrobiotic Approach*. Japan Publications. ISBN 087040-667-1.

Kushi, Michio; Kushi, Aveline; Esko, Edward; Esko, Wendy. (1986). *Macrobiotic Child Care and Family Health*. Japan Publications. ISBN 978-0870406126.

Kushi, Michio; Kushi, Aveline; Esko, Edward; Esko, Wendy. (1984). *Macrobiotic Pregnancy and Care of the Newborn*. Japan Publications. ISBN 978-0870405310.

Kushi, Michio; Jack, Alex (1985). *Diet for a Strong Heart*. St. Martin's Press. ISBN 0-312-20998-3.

Kushi, Michio; Kushi, Aveline; Jack, Alex (1985). *Macrobiotic Diet*. Japan Publications, revised 1993. ISBN 978-0870408786.

Porter, Jessica (2011). *The Hip Chick's Guide to Macrobiotics*. Avery Publications, ISBN 978-1583332054.

Waxman, Denny and Susan (2015). *The Complete Macrobiotic Diet*. Pegasus Books. ISBN 978-1605986661.

Yamamoto, Shizuko; McCarthy, Patrick (1979). *Barefoot Shiatsu*. Japan Publications. ISBN 978-0895298577.

History

* Kushi, Michio; Jack, Alex (2013). *The Book of Macrobiotics*. Square One Publications. ISBN 978-0-7570-0342-4.

Jack, Alex; Esko, Edward, editors (2015). *Remembering Michio*. Kushi Institute. ISBN 9781508852148.

Kotzsch, Ronald E. (1985). *Macrobiotics: Yesterday and Today*. Japan Publications. ISBN 978-0870406119.

*Kushi, Aveline; Jack, Alex (1988). *Aveline: The Life and the Dream of the Woman Behind Macrobiotics Today*. Japan Publications. ISBN 0-87040-693-0.

Mizuno Namboku (1807); translated by Kushi, Michio; Kushi, Aveline; Jack, Alex (1985). *Food Governs Your Destiny*. Japan Publications, 1992. ISBN 0-87040-788-0.

Tara, William(1985). *Macrobiotics and Human Behavior*. Japan Publications. ISBN 978-0870406027.

Philosophy and Science

*Kushi, Michio; Jack, Alex (2013). *The Book of Macrobiotics*. Square One Publications. ISBN 978-0-7570-0342-4.

Butler, Samuel (1870). *Erewhon*. New American Library, 1960.

Esko, Edward (2012). *Yin Yang Primer*. Amberwaves Press. ISBN 9781477645604.

Esko, Edward; Jack, Alex (2011). *Cool Fusion: A Quantum Solution to Peak Minerals, Nuclear Waste, and Future Metals Shock*. Amberwaves Press. ISBN 9781477563724.

Esko, Edward; Jack, Alex (2014). *Corking the Nuclear Genie*. Amberwaves Press. ISBN 9781493664740.

Ferré, Carl, ed. (2013). *Essential Ohsawa: From Food to Health, Happiness to Freedom*. George Ohsawa Macrobiotic Foundation. ISBN 978-0918860576.

*Hufeland, Christolph W., M.D. (1796). *Macrobiotics or the Art of Prolonging Life*.

*I Ching or Book of Changes (1950). Translated by Richard Wilhelm and Cary F. Baynes. Princeton University Press.

Kervran, Louis (1972). *Biological Transmutations*. George Ohsawa Macrobiotic Foundation, 2011 edition. ISBN 978-0918860651

*Kushi, Michio; Jack, Alex (1992). *The Gospel of Peace: Jesus's Teachings of Eternal Truth*. Japan Publications. ISBN 0-87040-797-X.

*Ohsawa, George (1931). *The Unique Principle*: *The Philosophy of Macrobiotics*. George Ohsawa Macrobiotic Foundation, 1973 edition. ISBN 978-0918860170.

Wang, Robin R. (2012). *Yinyang: The Way of Heaven and Earth in Chinese Thought and Culture*. Cambridge University Press. ISBN 9780521165136.

Periodicals

Amberwaves (2001-), Becket, Massachusetts
Macrobiotics Today (1984-), Oroville, California
Das Grosse Leben, Germany

About the Authors

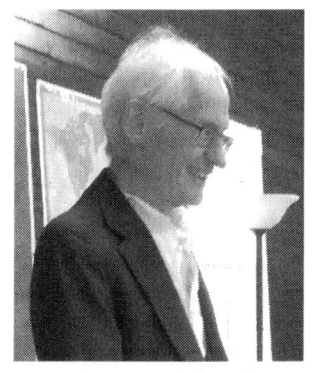

Alex Jack is president of Planetary Health and has served as executive director of Kushi Institute and editor-in-chief of *East West Journal*. He has helped introduce macrobiotics to China and Russia and has written many books with Michio and Aveline Kushi, including *The Cancer Prevention Diet*, *Aveline Kushi's Complete Guide to Macrobiotic Cooking*, *The Book of Macrobiotics*, and *One Peaceful World*. He is on the guest faculty of the Kushi Institute of Europe and has presented at the Cardiology Institute in St. Petersburg, the Zen Temple in Beijing, Shakespeare's New Globe Theatre in London, and Rosas Dance Company in Brussels. He is the founder of www.thecancerpreventiondiet.com.

Edward Esko is vice president of Planetary Health and has served as associate director of Kushi Institute, executive director of the East West Foundation, and founder of Quantum Rabbit LLC, a new technology company dedicated to a healthy and sustainable future. He is the author of *Contemporary Macrobiotics, Yin Yang Primer, Rice Field Essays, One Peaceful Universe,* and other books. He is the founder of Macrobiotic Classroom: www.macrobioticclassroom.com.

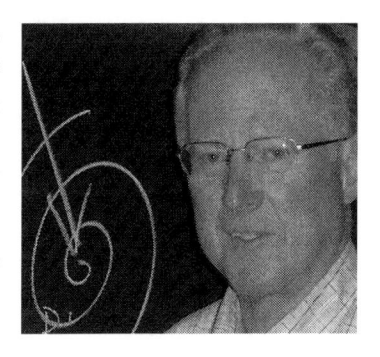

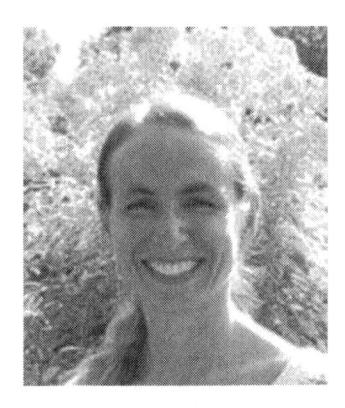

Bettina Zumdick is a teacher, counselor, humanitarian, and author who has integrated modern knowledge of the West with the ancient wisdom of the East. With a strong background in Food Science, Dietetics, and Nutrition from Wilhelms University in Muenster, Germany, she has shared her knowledge of food as medicine for over 30 years. Her experience in the fields of holistic health, wellness, and macrobiotics has helped thousands of people to regain and maintain their health and vibrancy. She is the author of *Authentic Foods* and founder of the Culinary Medicine School in Lee, Massachusetts. www.culinarymedicineschool.com.

References

[1] "Macrobiotic Diet," Wikipedia, www.wikipedia.com. Retrieved April 8, 2017. It is true that George Ohsawa wrote a popular book *Zen Macrobiotics* linking macrobiotics with Zen Buddhism. But the title was more in the cultural or avant garde sense of Zen Beatniks and awakening to a higher reality than identifying with the venerable religious tradition. In this dynamic little book, published in 1965 as the first wave of macrobiotics made an impression on America, Ohsawa contrasted *Shojin Ryori*, the elegant, spiritually refined cooking of the traditional Zen monastery, with the low, sensory food prepared in ordinary Chinese and Japanese restaurants. He made it clear that Zen was not the only, or major, historical stream contributing to modern macrobiotics. "It is because of the Macrobiotic teaching of Lao-tse, Sun Tzu Wu, Confucius, Buddha, Nagarjuna, the Shontoists, and long before them, the sages who produced the gret medical science of India, that millions of people in the Far East enjoyed happiness and freedom, culture and comparative peace for thousands of years. They, along with the ancient Greeks, knew that a sound, clear mind cannot exist in a tense, disturbed body" (pp. x, 1).

[2] Kushi, Michio (2013). *The Book of Macrobiotics*.

[3] Kuhn, Thomas S. (1962). *The Structure of Scientific Revolutions*,

[4] TruthWiki, "Wikipedia," retrieved April 7, 2017.

[5] Cohen, Noam. "A History Department Bans Citing Wikipedia as a Research Source," *New York Times*, Feb. 21, 2007.

[6] Wells, Patricia. "Marobiotics: A Principle Not a Diet," *New York Times*, July 19, 1978.

[7] *Dietary Guidelines for Americans, 2000*. U.S. Department of Health and Human Services and U.S. Department of Agriculture.

[8] "The Healing Power of a Heart-Healthy Diet," *Consumer Reports*, May 2017, p. 32.

[9] Kushi, Michio; Jack, Alex (2013). *The Book of Macrobiotics: The Universal Way to Health, Happiness, and Peace*. Square One Publications, pp. xii-xvii. ISBN 9780757004407.

[10] Kushi, Michio; Jack, Alex (2017). *One Peaceful World: Creating a Healthy and Harmonious Mind, Home, and World Community, pp.* xii-xvii. Square One Publications. ISBN 978-0-0-7570-0440-7.

[11] Individual studies are listed below.

[12] Kunz, Jeffrey R. M., and Finkel, Asher J., eds. (1987) *The American Medical Association Family Medical Guide*, Random House, p. 27. ISBN 0-394-55582-1.

[13] Smithsonian Institution Archives. http://siris-archives.si.edu/ipac20/ipac.jsp?profile=all&source.

[14] Hippocrates; Jones, William, translator. *Airs, Waters, Places*. Harvard University Press, 1923. Volume IV, p. 79. ISBN 978-0674991668.

[15] Kushi, Michio; Jack, Alex (2003). *The Macrobiotic Path to Total Health: A Complete Guide to Preventing and Relieving More Than 200 Chronic Conditions and Disorders Naturally*. Ballantine Books, p. 5. ISBN 0-345-43987-2.

[16] Shurtleff, William; Aoyagi, Akiko (2011). *History of Erewhon—Natural Foods Pioneer in the United States (1966-2011)*. ISBN: 978-1-928914-33-4.

[17] Gray, Sylvia Ruth (2016). *Eating Animals? Would George Ohsawa and Michio Kushi Be Vegan Today?* Amberwaves Press.

[18] "Zen Macrobiotic Diets". *JAMA: The Journal of the American Medical Association*. 218 (3):397. 1971. Doi:10.1001/jama.1971.03190160047009. "Simon, Beth Ann," *The Free Dictionary*. Christgau, Robert (1966). "Beth Ann and Microbioticism". "The Kosher of the Counterculture," *Time*. EBSCOhost. 96 (20). 16 November 1970.

[19] Stare, Frederick J. "The Diet That's Killing Our Kids," *Ladies Home Journal*. October, 1971, p. 70.

[20] *Dietary Goals for the United States* (1977), U.S. Senate Select Committee on Nutrition and Human Needs, second edition. https://naldc.nal.usda.gov/naldc/download.xhtml?id=1759572&content=PDF

[21] Brody, Jane. "Final Advice from Dr. Spock: Eat Only All Your Vegetables," *New York Times*, June 20, 1988.

[22] Spock, Benjamin, M.D; Parker, Charles (1998). *Dr. Spock's Baby and Child Care*. E. P. Dutton. ISBN 978-0525944171.

[23] See citations below for cancer, heart disease, etc.

[24] Kushi and Jack, *One Peaceful World,* passim.

[25] Macrobiotic Research Project," Jane Teas, Ph.D., principal investigator; Joan Cunningham, Ph.D., co-principal investigator, sponsored by the Centers for Disese Control.
Oct. 2000 to Sept 2002, University of South Carolina, Prevention Research Center, School of Public Health, Charleston SC. Minutes of the Fifth Meeting, Cancer Advisory Advisory Panel for Complementary and Alternative Medicine (CAPCAM), Bethesda, Maryland, February 25, 2002; Moss, Ralph, Ph.D. "The Olive Branch Bears Fruit," *The Moss Reports*, February 27, 2002. www.cancerdecisions.com/022702.html

[26] B. R. Goldin et al., "Effect of Diet on Excretion of Estrogens in Pre- and Postmenopausal Incidence of Breast Cancer in Vegetarian Women," *Cancer Research* 41:3771-73, 1981; Anthony J. Satillaro, M.D., *Recalled by Life: The Story of My Recovery from Cancer* with Tom Monte (Boston: Houghton-Mifflin, 1982); Office of Technology Assessment (OTA), *Unconventional Cancer Treatments*. Government Printing Office, 1990; James P. Carter et al., "Hypothesis: Dietary Management May Improve Survival from Nutritionally Linked Cancers Based on Analysis of Representative Cases," *Journal of the American College of Nutrition* 12:209-226, 1993; Franco Berrino et al., "Reducing Bioavailable Sex Hormones through a Comprehensive Change in Diet: the Diet and Androgens (DIANA) Randomized Trial," *Cancer Epidemiology, Biomarkers, & Prevention* 10: 25-33, January 2001; "Nutrition and Special Diet: Macrobiotics," M.D. Anderson Cancer Center, the University of Texas,www.mdanderson.org/departments/cime, 2003-2006; R. Kaaks, "Effects of Dietary Intervention on IGF-Binding Proteins, and Related Alterations in Sex Steroid Metabolism: The Diet and Androgens (DIANA) Randomized Trial," *European Journal of Clinical Nutrition* 57(9):1079-88, 2003; C. Colombo et al., "Plant-Based Diet, Serum Fatty Acid Profile, and Free Radicals in Postmenopausal Women: The Diet and Androgens (DIANA) Randomized Trial," *International Journal of Biological Markers* 20(3):169-76, 2005; G.A. Saxe et al., "Potential Attenuation of Disease Progression in Recurrent Prostate Cancer with Plant-Based Diet and Stress Reduction," *Integr Cancer Ther* 5(3)206-13, 2006; J.Y. Nguyen et al., "Adoption of a Plant-Based Diet by Patients with Recurrent Prostate Cancer," *Integr Cancer Ther* 5(3):214-23, 2006

[27] Jack, Alex (2002). *Biowisdom: A Natural Approach to Bioterrorism, Nuclear Radiation, GMOs, and Other Threats*. Amberwaves Press, pp. 8–17. ISBN 0-9708913-2-6.

[28] Kushi and Jack, *Macrobiotic Path*, p. viii.

[29] Ibid.

[30] Ibid.

[31] Congressional Record, V. 145, Pt. 8, May 24, 1999 to June 8 1999, 11812.

[32] Kushi and Jack. *Macrobiotic Path*, p. 15.

[33] Kushi and Jack, *Book of Macrobiotics*, pp. 11–25.

[34] Ibid, pp. 27–60.

[35] Kushi, Michio; Jack, Alex. *The Gospel of Peace: Jesus's Teachings of Eternal Truth.* Japan Publications, pp. 90–93. ISBN 0-87040-797-X.

[36] Kushi and Jack, *Gospel of Peace*, pp. 166–174.

[37] Kushi and Jack, *Book of Macrobiotics*, p. 19.

[38] Collins, Roy; Kerr, David (2001). "Etymology of the Word 'Macrobiotics' and Its Use in Modern Chinese Scholarship," *Sino-Platonic Papers,* Department of East Asian Languages and Civilizations University of Pennsylvania. www.sino-platonic.org.

[39] Kushi and Jack, *Gospel of Peace*, p. 55.

[40] Homer, *Iliad* 13.

[41] Kushi and Jack, *Book of Macrobiotics*, p. 20

[42] Hufeland, Christoph Wilhelm. [*Macrobiotic or the*] *Art of Prolonging Life*, 1797, edited by Erasmus Wilson (1854 edition), Arno Press, 1979, p. vii. ISBN 0-405-11817-1.

[43] Encyclopædia Americana (1838), Vol. 8, edited by Francis Lieber, Edward Wigglesworth.

[44] R. Burton, Richard (1856). *First Footsteps in East Africa.* J.M. Dutton, 1924 reprint, pp. 130–131.

[45] Lockyear, Norman (1909). *Nature* 79, p. 45. https://books.google.com/books

[46] Szekely, E. (1936); Weaver, L., tr., *Cosmos, Man and Society*. International Biogenic Society, p. 37.

[47] Toynbee, Arnold J. (1972). *A Study of History*. Oxford University Press, p. 89.

[48] Needham, Joseph (1974). *Science and Civilisation in China*, Cambridge University Press, Vol. 5, Pt 2, p.II

[49] Kaibara, Ekiken (1713). *Yojokun: Japanese Secret of Good Health*. Tokuma Shoten, 1974.

[50] Mizuno, Namboku (1807). *So Ho Goku Syu Shin Roku*. Published in English as *Food Governs Your Destiny: The Teachings of Namboku Mizuno*, translated by Michio and Aveline Kushi with Alex Jack. Japan Publications, 1991. ISBN 0-87040-788-0.

[51] Ishizuka, Sagen (1897). *Kagakuteki Shoku-Yo* ("A Chemical Nutritional Theory of Long Life"), Nippon C.I., 1975, and *Shokumotsu Yojoho: Ichimei Kagakuteki Shoku-Yo Tai Shin Ron* ("A Method for Nourishing Life Through Food: A Unique Chemical Food-Nourishment Theory of Body and Mind"), 1898. Nippon C.I., 1974.

[52] Ohsawa, George; Dufty, William (1965). *You Are All Sanpaku*. Citadel (1998 reprint). ISBN 978-0806507286.

[53] Kotzsch, Ronald, Ph.D. (1985). *Macrobiotics: Yesterday and Today*. Japan Publications. ISBN 978-0870406119.

[54] Sherman Goldman, "Statement of Purpose," *East West Journal*, 1974-1982.

[55] Kushi and Jack, *Macrobiotic Path*, p. 5.

[56] Kushi and Jack, *Book of Macrobiotics*, pp. 78–79.

[57] Kushi, Aveline; Jack, Alex (1985). *Aveline Kushi's Complete Guide to Macrobiotic Cooking*. Warner. ISBN 978-0446386340

[58] Kushi and Jack, *Book of Macrobiotics*, pp. 171-172.

[59] Book of Daniel 1: 8–17. Douay-Rheims American Edition, 1899.

[60] Kushi and Jack, *Macrobiotic Path*, p. 5

[61] Select Committee on Nutrition and Human Needs, U.S. Senate (1977). *Dietary Goals for the United States*. U.S. Government Printing Office.

[62] Bergan, J. G.; Brown, P. T. "Nutritional Status of 'New' Vegetarians," *Journal of the American Dietetic Association* 76:151-55, 1980.

[63] Hinds, Alison, BSc. "A Short Study of the Macrobiotic Diet." Queen Elizabeth College, University of London, 1985.

[64] Campbell, Ph.D., T. Colin Campbell; Campbell II, Thomas M. (2004, revised 2017), *The China Study*. Benbella Books.

[65] Harmon, Brook E. et al. (2015). "Nutrient Composition and Anti-inflammatory Potential of a Pre-scribed Macrobiotic Diet," *Nutrition and Cancer*, DOI: 10.1080/01635581.2015. 1055369

[66] Smith, Michael, M.D. (2017). "Macrobiotic Diet," Web MD, www.webmd.com. Retrieved March 27, 2017.

[67] Sacks, F. M.; Rosner, Bernard; Kass, Edward H. "Blood Pressure in Vegetarians," *American Journal of Epidemiology* 100:390-98, 1974.

[68] Sacks, F. M. et al. "Plasma Lipids and Lipoproteins in Vegetarians and Controls," *New England Journal of Medicine* 292:1148-51, 1975.

[69] *Healthy People: The Surgeon General's Report on Health Promotion and Disease Prevention*. Government Printing Office, 1979.

[70] Sacks, F. M. et al. "Effects of Ingestion of Meat on Plasma Cholesterol of Vegetarians," *Journal of the American Medical Association* 246:640-44, 1981.

[71] Castelli, William P. "Summary of Lessons from the Framingham Heart Study," Framingham, Mass., September, 1983.

[72] Kushi, Michio; Jack, Alex (1985). *Diet for a Strong Heart*. St. Martin's Press, p. 131. ISBN 978-0312304584

[73] Kohler, Jean; Kohler, Marie Ann (1979). *Healing Miracles from Macrobiotics*. Parker Publishing.

[74] Jack and Kushi, *Cancer Prevention Diet*, pp. 403–404.

[75] Dobic, Milenka (2000). *My Beautiful Life*. Avery Publishing. ISBN 978-1899171132.

[76] Benedict, Dirk (1991). Confessions of a Kamikaze Cowboy. Avery. ISBN 978-0895294791

[77] Nussbaum, Elaine (1992). *Recovery: From Cancer to Health Through Macrobiotics*. Japan Publications. ISBN 978-0870406430.

[78] Kushi and Jack, *The Cancer Prevention Diet*, pp. 430–431. St. Martin's Press. ISBN 9780312561062.

[79] *One Peaceful World Journal*, #6 August 1990.
[80] Satillaro, Anthony J., M.D.; Monte, Tom (1982). *Recalled by Life: The Story of My Recovery from Cancer*, Houghton-Mifflin, 1982.
[81] Kushi and Jack, *Cancer-Prevention Diet*, p. 351.
[82] Brown, Virginia, R.N.; Stayman, Susan (1982). Macrobiotic Miracle: How a Vermont Family Overcame Cancer. Japan Publications. ISBN 978-0870405730.
[83] The East West Foundation and Ann Fawcett (1992). *Cancer-Free: 30 Who Triumphed Over Cancer Naturally*. Japan Publications. ISBN 978-0870407949.
[84] Kushi and Jack, *Cancer-Prevention Diet*, pp. 313–314. *One Peaceful World Journal* #5, Spring, 1991.
[85] Geismar, Erin, "Montauk Man Still Cancer-Free After 6 Years," *East Hampton Press*, March 2, 2010.
[86] NIH Best Cases Study. University of South Carolina, Prevention Research Center, 2002.
[87] Minutes of the Fifth Meeting, Cancer Advisory Panel for Complementary and Alternative Medicine (CAPCAM), Bethesda, Maryland, February 25, 2002; Ralph Moss, Ph.D., "The Olive Branch Bears Fruit," *The Moss Reports*, February 27, 2002. www.cancerdecisions. com/022702.html
[88] Macrobiotic Research Project," Jane Teas, Ph.D., principal investigator; Joan Cunningham, Ph.D., co-principal investigator, sponsored by the Centers for Disease Control, October 2000 to September 2002, University of South Carolina, Prevention Research Center, School of Public Health, Charleston, S.C. www.macro-biotics.sph.sc.edu/project.htm
[89] "Nutrition and Special Diet: Macrobiotics," M.D. Anderson Cancer Center, the University of Texas,www.mdanderson.org/depart ments/cime, 2003-2006.
[90] B. R. Goldin et al. "Effect of Diet on Excretion of Estrogens in Pre- and Postmenopausal Incidence of Breast Cancer in Vegetarian Women," *Cancer Research* 41:3771-73, 1981.
[91] Teas, J; Harbison, M. L.; Gelman, R.S. (1984). "Dietary Seaweed [*Laminaria*] and Mammary Carcinogenesis in Rats, Cancer Research 44:2758-61.
[92] Yamamoto; Ichiro; et al. (1987). "The Effect of Dietary Seaweeds on 7,12-Dimethyl-Benz[a]Anthracene-Induced Mammary Tumorigenesis in Rats," *Cancer Letters* 35:109–18.
[93] Berrino, Franco et al. "Reducing Bioavailable Sex Hormones through a Comprehensive Change in Diet: the Diet and Androgens (DIANA) Randomized Trial," *Cancer Epidemiology, Biomarkers, & Prevention* 10: 25-33, January 2001.
[94] Allen, N.E. et al. "The associations of diet with serum insulin-like growth factor I and its main binding proteins in 292 women meat-eaters, vegetarians, and vegans. *Cancer Epidemiol Biomarkers Prev.* 2002;11(11):1441-1448.
[95] Nkondjock, A. et al. "Diet Quality and BRCA-associated breast cancer risk," Breast Cancer Res Treat. 2007 Jul;103(3):361-9. 84 Nkondjock A. et al., "Diet, lifestyle and BRCA-related breast cancer risk among French-Canadians," *Breast Cancer Res Treat*. 2006 Aug;98(3):285-94. Ghadirian P., et al., "Breast cancer risk in relation to the joint effect of BRCA mutations and diet diversity," *Breast Cancer Res Treat*. 2009 Sep;117(2):417-22.
[96] Jernstrom, H. et al., "Breast-feeding and the risk of breast cancer in BRCA1 and BRCA2 mutation carriers," *Journal National Cancer Institute*, 2004;96(14):1094-1098.
13. Cho E, Spiegelman D, Hunter DJ, et al. Premenopausal fat intake and risk of breast cancer. *J Natl Cancer Inst*. 95:1079-85, 2003.
14. "High-Fat Dairy Products Linked to Poorer Breast Cancer Survival," Kaiser Permanente, Press Release, March 14, 2013.
[99] Jack, Alex et al. (2013). *Nutrition vs. Surgery: The Breast Cancer Controversy*, p. 3–10. Amberwaves Press.
[100] Barillari, J. et al. "Kaiware Daikon (*Raphanus sativus* L.) extract: a naturally multipotent chemopreventive agent," *J Agric Food Chem*. 2008 Sep 10;56(17):7823-30.
[101] Ollberding, N.J. et al. "Legume, soy, tofu, and isoflavone intake and endometrial cancer risk in postmenopausal women in the multiethnic cohort study," *J Natl Cancer Inst* 2012 Jan4:104(1):67-76.
[102] A. Nakamura et al. "Genistein inhibits cell invasion and motility by inducing cell differentiation in murine osteosarcoma cell line LM8, *BMC Cell Biol*. 2012 Sep 26;13:24.

[103] Carter, James P. et al. "Hypothesis: Dietary Management May Improve Survival from Nutritionally Linked Cancers Based on Analysis of Representative Cases," *Journal of the American College of Nutrition* 12:209-226, 1993.

[104] Ibid.

[105] Saxe, G.A. et al. "Potential Attenuation of Disease Progression in Recurrent Prostate Cancer with Plant-Based Diet and Stress Reduction," *Integr Cancer Ther* 5(3)206-13, 2006.

[106] Hirayama, T. "Relationship of Soybean Paste Soup Intake to Gastric Cancer Risk," *Nutrition and Cancer* 3: 223–33.

[107] Chihara, G. et al. "Fractionation and Purification of the Polysaccharides with Marked Antitumor Activity, Especially Lentinan, from *Lentinus edodes* (Berk.) Sing. (An Edible Mushroom), *Cancer Research* 30: 2776–81.

[108] "Complementary and Alternative Therapies, American Cancer Society Internet Site, 1997; "Alternative and Complementary Therapies," *Cancer* 77(6), 1996.

[109] "Guide for Nutrition and Physical Activity for Cancer Survivors," *CA: A Cancer Journal for Clinicians*, Sept-Oct. 2003.

[110] American Cancer Society guidelines on nutrition and physical activity for cancer prevention (2012), Lawrence H. Kushi ScD. CA: *A Cancer Journal for Clinicians* Volume 62, Issue 1 January/February 2012. Pages 30–67.

[111] Sadovsky, Richard. "Complementary and Alternative Medical Therapies for Cancer," *American Family Physician*, May 1, 2003.

[112] American Cancer Society (2012), op cit.

[113] "Patients with Kaposi Sarcoma Who Opt for No Treatment," Letter. *Lancet*, July 1985.

[114] Kushi, Michio; Jack (1995). *AIDS and Beyond: Dietary and Lifestyle Guidelines for New Viral and Bacterial Disease.* One Peaceful World Press. (1997) *Humanity at the Crossroads.* One Peaceful Word Press. (2003) *Macrobiotic Path to Total Health.*

[115] "Umeboshi Have H1N1 Suppressant," *Japan Times,* June 3, 2010.

[116] Hafstraim, I. et al. "A Vegan Diet Free of Gluten Improves the Symptoms of Rheumatoid Arthritis," *Rheumatology* 40(10):1175-79, 2001.

[117] McDougall, John. "Diet: The Only Real Hope for Arthritis*,*" *The McDougall Newsletter*, May/June, 1998.

[118] Childers, N. F.; Margoles, M. S. "An Apparent Relation of Nightshades (Solanaceae) to Arthritis," *Journal of Neurological and Orthopedic Medical Surgery* 12:227-231, 1993.

[119] Campbell, Don (1997). *The Mozart Effect.* Avon Books.

[120] Harvey, Judy. "Overcoming Autism with Diet," *One Peaceful World Journal* 29:1, Winter 1997.

[121] Anonymous. *Macrobiotic Recovery from Autism,* Planetary Health/Amberwaves, 2014.

[122] Knivsber, A. M. et al. "Reports on Dietary Intervention in Autistic Disorders," *Nutri Neurosci* (4)1:25-37, 2001. A. M. Knivsber et al., "A Randomized Study of Dietary Intervention in Autistic Syndrome," *Nutr Neurosci* 5(4):251-61, 2002.

[123] Jack, Alex. "The Origin of Celiac," *Amberwaves Journal*, Spring 2014.

[124] Ventura, Valerie. "A Comparative Study of the Meals Provided for Pre-School Children by Two Day Nurseries," Department of Nutrition, Queen Elizabeth College, 1980.

[125] Shull, M. W. et al. "Velocities of Growth in Vegetarian Preschool Children," *Pediatrics* 60:410-17, 1977.

[126] Dwyer, J. T. et al. "Mental Age and I.Q. of Predominantly Vegetarian Children," *Journal of the American Dietetic Association* 76:142-47, 1980.

[127] Esko, Edward; Jack, Alex; and Harper, Virginia. *Crohn's and Colitis: The Macrobiotic Approach*, Amberwaves Press, 2016.

[128] Bhjumisawasdi, J. et al. "The Self-Reliant System for Alternative Care of Diabetes Mellitus Patients—Experience Macrobiotic Management in Trad Province," *Journal of the Medical Association of Thailand* 89(12):2104-15, 2006.

[129] Porrata, Carmen, M.D., PhD., et al. "Ma-Pi 2 Macrobiotic Diet Intervention in Adults with Type 2 Diabetes Mellitus," *MEDICC Review*, Fall 2009, 11(4):29-35.

[130] Hu, Emily A. et al. "White rice consumption and risk of type 2 diabetes: meta-analysis and system-

atic review, *BMJ* 2012; 344.

[131] Lerman, Robert H., M.D., Ph.D. "The Macrobiotic Diet in Chronic Disease," *Nutri Clin Prac* December 2010; 25(6):621-626.

[132] Jack, Alex; Esko, Edward (2014). *Ebola & Diet.* Planetary Health, Inc., Michio Kushi with the Kushi Institute Research and Faculty Committee, *Ebola Relief and Prevetion: Dieary Recommendations and Proposals.* Kushi Institute, 2014. www.ebolaanddiet.com

[133] Rogers, Sherry A. M.D. "From HEAL's Advisory Board: The Cure Is in the Kitchen—One Case History," *The Human Ecologist*, Fall 1990, pp. 19-21.

[134] Rogers, Sherry A., M.D. "Improvement in Chemical Sensitivity with the Macrobiotic Diet," *Journal of Applied Nutrition* 48: 85-92, 1996.

[135] Lieff, Jonathan et al. (1987). "Study Results of Dietary Change in Shattuck Hospital Geropsychiatric Wards, 5 North and 6 North," in Michio Kushi, *Crime and Diet*, pp. 229-34.

[136] Green, Peter (2010). *Celiac Disease: A Hidden Epidemic.* William Morrow. ISBN 978-0060766948.

[137] Thomas, Katya. "I Love Gluten," *Amberwaves Journal*, Autumn 2012.

[138] Iglehart, Tom (1987). "The Shattuck Model: Macrobiotics in an Institution," in Michio Kushi et al., *Crime and Diet*. Japan Publications, 1987, pp. 203-29. ISBN 978-0870406829.

[139] Armelin, Cecilia. "Wholefood Diet," National Children's Hospital, Dublin, Ireland, 1989.

[140] Wetzel, Miriam S. et al. "Courses Involving Complementary and Alternative Medicine at U.S. Medical Schools." *Journal of the American Medical Association* 280:784-87, 1998.

[141] "Most medical schools offer courses in alternative medicine." Vox.com, July 8, 2015.

[142] Briscoe, David; Mahoney-Briscoe, Charlotte (1989). *A Personal Peace: Macrobiotic Reflections on Mental and Emotional Recovery: Macrobiotic Reflections on Mental and Emotional Recovery.* Japan Publications. ISBN 978-0870406980.

[143] Harnish, Stephen, M.D. (1989). "On My Awakening to the Macrobiotic Way," *Doctors Look at Macrobiotics*. Japan Publications. ISBN 978-0870406867.

[144] Blanc, Bernard H.; Hertel, Hans U. "Influence on Man: Comparative Study About Food Prepared Conventionally and in the Microwave Oven," *Raum & Zeit*, 3(2): 1992.

[145] Farrell, H.V. (1988). "PMS Is Not PMS," *Doctors Look at Macrobiotics*, pp. 177-91.

[146] Akizuki, Tatsuichiro, M.D. *Nagasaki 1945* (1980). Quartet Books, 1981. Akizuki, Tatsuichiro, M.D., "How We Survived Nagasaki," *East West Journal*, December 1980.

[147] Furo, Hiroko, Ph.D. "Dietary Practices of Hiroshima/Nagasaki Atomic Bomb Survivors," Illinois Wesleyan University, 2006.

[148] Skoryna, S.C. et al. "Studies on Inhibition of Intestinal Absorption of Radioactive Strontium," *Canadian Medical Association Journal* 91: 285-88, 1964.

[149] "Miso Shows Promise as Treatment for Radiation," *Japan Times*, September 27, 1988.

[150] Jack, Alex. "Soviets Embrace Macrobiotics," *One Peaceful World* 6:1 Autumn/Winter, 1990.

[151] "Effects of agar (kanten) diet on obese patients with impaired glucose tolerance and type 2 diabetes," *Diabetes, Obesity, and Metabolism*, 7(1):40–46, 2005.

[152] Ikeda, Y. et al. "Intake of Fermented Soybeans, Natto, Is Associated with Reduced Bone Loss in Postmenopausal Women: Japanese Population-Based Osteoporosis (JPOS) Study," J Nutri 136(5):1323-8, 2006.

[153] Cardini, F.; Weixin, H. "Moxibustion for correction of breech presentation: a randomized controlled trial," *JAMA*. 1998 Nov 11;280(18):1580-4.

[154] Coyle, M. E. et al. "Cephalic version by moxibustion for breech presentation," *Cochrane Database Syst Rev*. 2012 May 16;(5):CD003928.

[155] Amir, N. et al. "Efficacy comparison between Chinese medicine's labor inducement methods and conventional methods customary in hospitals," Harefuah. 2015 Jan;154(1):47-51, 67, 66.

[156] Jack, Alex; Jack, Gale (2006). *Chewing Made Easy: 42 Benefits, Tips, and Techniques.* Macrobiotic Path.

[157] "The Veggie Baseball Team," *Parade Magazine*, April 15, 1984.

[158] Walsh, Michael. "Sounds of Silence," *Time*, June 24, 2001.

[159] "Bushmen," NationalGeographic.com, January 2000.

[160] Richards, M.P. "A Brief Review of the Archaeological Evidence for Palaeolithic and Neolithic Subsistence," *Eur J Clin Nutri* 2002 Dec;56(12):1262-78.

[161] Wrangham, Richard (2009). *Catching Fire: How Cooking Made Us Human.* Basic Books 2009.

[162] "Diet likely changed game for some hominids 3.5 million years ago," ScienceDaily.com, June 13, 2013. *Proceedings of the National Academy of Sciences*, June 3, 2013.

[163] Ferran Estebaranz, et al. "Buccal dental microwear analyses support greater specialization in consumption of hard foodstuffs for *Australopithecus anamensis*." *Journal of Anthropological Sciences*, 2012; 90: 1-24.

[164] Mercader, Julio, "Mozambican Grass Seed Consumption During the Middle Stone Age," *Science* 326:Dec. 18, 2009. www.sciencemag.org.

[165] Fairservis, Walter Ashlin (1975). *The Threshold of Civilization: An Experiment in Prehistory*. Charles Scribner's Sons.

[166] "The Stone Age baker: Cavemen 'ate bread, not just meat.'" *Daily Mail Reporter*, October 19, 2010.

[167] *Amberwaves Journal* 2001-2017.

[168] Jack, Alex (2000). *Imagine a World Without Monarch Butterflies: Awakening to the Hazards of Genetically Altered Foods*, foreword by Congressman Dennis J. Kucinich. One Peaceful World Press. ISBN 9781882984398.

[169] Cummins, Joseph (2001). "The First Independent Study of Genetically Engineered LibertyLink Rice," www.amberwaves.org.

[170] Schoenthaler, S., Ph.D. "The Effect of Sugar on the Treatment and Control of Antisocial Behavior," *International Journal of Biosocial Research* 3(1):1-9, 1982.

[171] Seaker, Meg. "Fighting Crime with Diet: Report from a Portuguese Prison," *East West Journal*, July, 1982, pp. 26-34.

[172] Jack, Alex (2002). *Sex, Lies, and GMOs*, Amberwaves Press.

[173] Kushi and Jack, *One Peaceful World*, pp. 28–31.

[174] Kushi and Jack, *One Peaceful World*, pp. 38–39.

[175] "Bringing Brown Rice and Peace to Syria," *Amberwaves Journal*, Summer 2012.

[176] Kushi and Jack, *One Peaceful World*, pp. 75–77.

[177] Jack, Alex. "Nutrition Under Siege," *One Peaceful World Journal* 34:1, 7–9, 1998.

[178] *Livestock's Long Shadow*, UN Food & Agricultural Organization, 2006.

[179] Eishel, Gidon; Martin Pamela. "Study: vegan diets healthier for planet, people than meat diets," *Earth Interactions*, April 2006.

[180] Loladze, I (2014). "Hidden shift of the ionome of plants exposed to elevated CO2 depletes minerals at the base of human nutrition." elife. 2014 3:e02245 http://www.researchgate.net/profile/Irakli_Loladze

[181] "Mobile Phones Could Lead to Bee Decline, *The Ecologist*, April 2007.

[182] "Cell Phones," National Toxicology Program, last modified Sep. 13, 2016, http://ntp.niehs.nih.gov/results/areas/cellphones/. "Cell Phone Radiation Boos Cancer Rates in Animals; $25 Million NTP Study Finds Brain Tumors," *Microwave News*, May 25, 2016. "ACS Responds to New Study Linking Cell Phone Radiation to Cancer," American Cancer Society, May 2017, http://pressroomcancer.org/NTP2016.

[183] Kervran, Louis C. (1972). *Biological Transmutations*, Swan House.

[184] Kushi, Michio; Esko, Edward (1994). *The Philosopher's Stone*. One Peaceful World Press.

[185] Goldfein, Solomon. "Energy Development from Elemental Transmutations in Biological Systems," Report 2247, Ft. Belvoir, Va.: U.S. Army Mobility Equipment Research and Development Command, 1978.

[186] Esko, Edward; Jack, Alex (2011). *Cool Fusion: A Quantum Solution to Peak Minerals, Nuclear Waste and Future Metal Shock*. Amberwaves Press. ISBN 978-1477563724.

[187] Falchi et al. The new world atlas of artificial night sky brightness," *Sci. Adv.* 2016;2.

[188] Jack, Alex. "A Dark Starless World," *Amberwaves Journal,* Autumn 2016.

[189] Kushi and Jack, *Book of Macrobiotics*, p. 4.

Special thanks to Sachi Kato, Nancy Adler, and other photographers for use of their wonderful pictures and graphics.

Printed in Great Britain
by Amazon